Knowing COVID-19

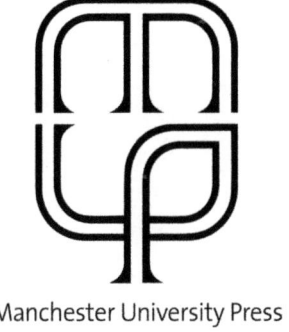

Manchester University Press

Knowing COVID-19

The pandemic and beyond

Edited by

Fred Cooper and Des Fitzgerald

MANCHESTER UNIVERSITY PRESS

Copyright © Manchester University Press 2024

While copyright in the volume as a whole is vested in Manchester University Press, copyright in individual chapters belongs to their respective authors, and no chapter may be reproduced wholly or in part without the express permission in writing of both author and publisher.

An electronic version has been made freely available under a Creative Commons (CC BY) licence, which permits commercial use, distribution and reproduction provided the author(s) and Manchester University Press are fully cited. Details of the licence can be viewed at https://creativecommons.org/licenses/by/4.0/

This work was supported by the Arts and Humanities Research Council.

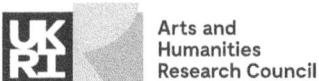

Published by Manchester University Press
Oxford Road, Manchester, M13 9PL

www.manchesteruniversitypress.co.uk

British Library Cataloguing-in-Publication Data
A catalogue record for this book is available from the British Library

ISBN 978 1 5261 7864 0 hardback

First published 2024

The publisher has no responsibility for the persistence or accuracy of URLs for any external or third-party internet websites referred to in this book, and does not guarantee that any content on such websites is, or will remain, accurate or appropriate.

Typeset by Newgen Publishing UK

Contents

Series preface: The pandemic and beyond – Pascale Aebischer, Fred Cooper, Des Fitzgerald, Karen Gray, Caroline Redhead, Melanie Smallman and Victoria Tischler — vii
List of figures — xxv
Contributors — xxvii

Introduction – Knowing COVID-19: The pandemic and beyond – Fred Cooper and Des Fitzgerald — 1

1. Pandemic imaginaries of interspecies relatedness: More-than-human microbial methods on the bus – Charlotte Veal, Paul Hurley, Emma Roe and Sandra Wilks — 16
2. Deafblindness, touch and COVID-19 – Azadeh Emadi — 41
3. Testing, testing: What about the instructions? – Sue Walker, Josefina Bravo and Al Edwards — 60
4. Home and neighbourhood: Pandemic geographies of dwelling and belonging – Alison Blunt, Kathy Burrell, Georgina Endfield, Miri Lawrence, Eithne Nightingale, Alastair Owens, Jacqueline Waldock and Annabelle Wilkins — 86
5. Crisis and engagement: The emotional toll of museum work during the COVID-19 pandemic – Elizabeth Crooke and David Farrell-Banks — 113
6. Storying older women's immobilities and gender-based violence in the COVID-19 pandemic – Lesley Murray, Amanda Holt and Jessica Moriarty — 136

7 Empowering obstinate memory: The experiences of Black, Asian and migrant nurses before and during the pandemic – Anandi Ramamurthy and Ken Fero   156

8 The shameful dead: Vaccine hesitancy, shame and necropolitics during COVID-19 – Fred Cooper, Luna Dolezal and Arthur Rose   179

Index   202

Series preface: The pandemic and beyond

Pascale Aebischer, Fred Cooper, Des Fitzgerald, Karen Gray, Caroline Redhead, Melanie Smallman and Victoria Tischler

In the first days of 2020, the coronavirus (COVID-19) pandemic began to spread across the globe. It prompted a concerted international research effort which set out to understand not just the workings of the virus, but the ways that we responded to, lived and died with it. This led to a significant body of work being produced at speed, in which arts and humanities played a crucial role. In the UK, *The Pandemic and Beyond: The Arts and Humanities Contribution to Covid Research and Recovery* was established by the Arts and Humanities Research Council (AHRC) early in 2021 to coordinate this research effort.[1] Over the span of two years, *The Pandemic and Beyond* grew into a virtual hub that enabled over seventy COVID-19 research teams funded by the AHRC to meet, exchange ideas and work together to ensure that their research would make a difference on the ground.[2]

This series is a legacy of this collaboration and bears witness to an extraordinary period, in which arts and humanities research became an integral part of the UK's research response to an emergency, leading to tangible changes in the role, purpose and methods of the arts and humanities, and laying important human foundations for recovery. It is divided into four volumes, each corresponding to four research clusters co-produced during the coordination process. A first group focused on working with professionals and policymakers in the creative industries to investigate the existential struggles of creative workers and organisations impacted by the ban on live in-person performance, and to devise new ways of connecting people through live arts while trying to build more inclusive and sustainable industry structures. A second set of research teams connected arts and creative practitioners with cultural and community organisations, as well as care settings, with whom they worked to alleviate the social and mental health impacts of public health restrictions. These projects drew on arts- and nature-based activities to forge pathways for improving mental and physical health for individuals and communities. A third cluster examined the informational and epistemic experience of a pandemic that was a whirlwind of often deeply confusing and contested data. Artists, designers and linguists explored design solutions and devised how public health messages could be formulated so that they would reach the communities most severely affected by the spread of the virus. A final group of researchers concentrated on scrutinising legislation and guidance issued in haste, and grappled with thorny questions of rights and responsibilities, seeking to underpin developing scientific understanding with values-based frameworks that offered a more nuanced approach to balancing risks and benefits.

The richness of this research portfolio stems not only from its breadth but also from the ingenuity of the teams involved, members of which rapidly applied their expertise and creativity to a problem few had foreseen, working with communities whose vulnerabilities and prior marginalisation had been exacerbated disproportionately by the pandemic (Ryan, 2022: 198). What was initially perceived principally as a public health crisis was impacting on the population in myriad ways that branched well beyond physical health; encompassing mental health, but also social cohesion, cross-generational justice, trust in governance, and economic distress. Looking back over the first few years of the pandemic, the authors of a report for the Higher Education Policy Institute (HEPI) conclude that the 'pandemic was a watershed moment for the Humanities because the importance of the variety and quality of individual human experience rose to the surface in our collective re-evaluation of priorities' (Thain et al., 2023: 13). Arts and humanities research concentrated on the human impacts of the crises that intersected in this moment, working to resolve them, mitigate harms and examine some of the most fundamental human questions across macro and micro crisis contexts, from the national and international to the local and hyper-local. As these volumes show, this work was characterised by cross-fertilisation between disciplines and an emphasis on partnership working. It featured collaboration; between academic and public institutions, but also, notably, with community groups and frontline organisations, such as those representing health and social care. Collaborations also extended to industry, and regional, sectoral and national policymakers. We know from analysis of surveys of those involved in *Pandemic and Beyond* research that for many this involved drawing on existing relationships, which deepened and strengthened as the fluctuations of the pandemic necessitated constant dialogue and increased accountability on all sides (Aebischer et al., 2022: 26–29). For others, the pandemic resulted in potentially fruitful new connections, and the promise of further research, work that continues to be relevant and have impacts on policy and practice.

All of this required new ways of working, and the ability to reconcile the theoretically conceptualised and deliberative methodologies associated with humanities research, which often take years to mature into publication, with quick and direct application, which often left little scope for fine calibration and reflective writing. The temporal demand for research outputs, and their new or altered audiences, exerted intense and immediate demands on researchers. Policymakers expressed an appetite for actionable findings to support decision-making, and frontline workers, while exhausted and short of time and resources, were desperate for support; research, in consequence, was predominantly pragmatic and focused on solutions. This meant a sometimes uneasy pivot to new ways of working and new modalities and timescales for doing and sharing work. Researchers did not always find it easy to reach those for whom their findings might have been most relevant, but many published policy briefings or held private meetings to share their insights and recommendations with potential user groups. Some projects embedded researchers within policy or service delivery organisations, narrowing the gap between research and practice still further. Work was often cyclical or iterative, with results shared earlier and more frequently, for example through pre-prints or the release of preliminary findings; if not a direct prerequisite for funding, the word 'rapid' in the UK Research and Innovation (UKRI) COVID-19 call certainly implied that researchers had to reconsider how and when in the life cycle of a project potentially significant knowledge was shared. There was a flowering of online engagement and dissemination as research was translated into a rich variety of deeply practical resources. These included frameworks for action, advice for public health messaging, interventions that responded to real-time problems such as the isolation of residents and staff in care homes or the design of personal protective equipment (PPE), and co-producing guidance for employers of artists performing in digital live shows from their homes.

As *Pandemic and Beyond* researchers explored the dynamic nature of individual and collective experiences of the pandemic, they also demonstrated a particular sensitivity to those for whom its effects have been felt unequally, and for whom suffering has been most profound. Readers will find this concern consistently exemplified throughout these volumes. Indeed, our brief to the authors in this series invited them to create a space where those voices could be part of the conversation. Such work was by no means easy to do. It was ethically complex, requiring heightened reflexivity and cultural competency. It was complicated by the requirements for social distancing and the need to prioritise the safety and wellbeing of both participants and researchers. As one research leader put it: 'you cannot build diversity into a project from scratch under these conditions' (Aebischer et al., 2022: 27).

Carrying out research during a pandemic necessitated innovation and adaptation at all levels. This is reflected in the research methods adopted: mixed, interdisciplinary and often participatory or arts-based, with projects bringing immediate benefits to participants and communities even as policymakers were targeted with written work. In many of the projects, more reflective and long-form modes of writing were either not part of the research design or postponed to a later date, to allow for retrospective analysis and evaluation. Meanwhile, the nascent field of arts and health was propelled to the foreground by the pandemic. A growing evidence base demonstrates the importance of multiple artistic modalities (including music, visual art, poetry and drama) in supporting health and wellbeing for a range of physical and mental health conditions. In these contexts, research by *Pandemic and Beyond* teams was able to highlight the vital role of artistic and creative practice through exposing the dangerousness of working conditions for frontline staff, including for the predominantly female workforce in social care settings. Arts-based projects were able to offer practical tools and emotional support for care workers, while helping to alleviate the isolation that many felt when confined to their homes by re-creating artistic activities that were delivered via post, online or outdoors. With remarkable speed, researchers working with arts and cultural providers pivoted to developing suitable resources and freely shared their work with collaborators and user groups.

At times, however, things moved frustratingly slowly, while structures around the research (including university recruitment, facilities, ethics and funding) creaked and failed to keep up; at other times, the most fundamental changes and compromises to research design had to be made at speed, to respond to events as they happened. When this research was at its best, there were refreshingly democratic opportunities for everyone involved to learn and apply new skills and take on new responsibilities. At their worst, however, the conditions in which research was conducted during the pandemic replicated existing structural problems in the academy. A great deal of the work was done by early career researchers on short-term contracts, for example, and researchers found themselves giving more than their contracted hours to this work, alongside their commitments to delivering newly remote or hybrid teaching, often while caring for home-schooled children or dealing with the impacts of the pandemic on their own networks and home environments. While it was often deeply rewarding, many researchers, like others in the population generally, found the lack of a distinction between home, work and the stresses of pandemic life difficult to negotiate. Remote working proved methodologically, physically and mentally challenging. However, as these chapters demonstrate so clearly, it led to the rapid creation and deployment of new tools and technologies for data collection, analysis and collaboration. These, in turn, are exerting pressure on funders and policymakers in UK Higher Education to adapt their frameworks to recognise the value and complexity of this type of crisis- and solutions-oriented collaborative response in arts and humanities research.

The work presented in this series as a distinctive and coherent portfolio is, of course, just part of a much wider programme of research to mitigate the effects of the pandemic and to address the COVID-19 emergency that was funded through UKRI.[3] While the projects within the *Pandemic and Beyond* portfolio were all designed, in line with the parameters of the original rapid-response funding call, to take a largely UK focus, a range of other projects and funding calls cast their gaze further afield.

For some existing projects with an international focus, this 'created new opportunities for exploration of existing topics' that were exacerbated by the pandemic (Pirgova-Morgan, 2022: 27). Other schemes which are not represented in these volumes, for instance the UKRI Global Research Challenges/Newton Fund, brought together researchers in the UK and in low- and middle-income countries. More than forty such collaborative projects sought to gain insights and provide support during the pandemic, including projects aiming to improve engagement with COVID-19 public health messages to develop online psychological support through the arts in Rwanda; and to find ways of engaging vulnerable communities in Brazil on the consequences of the pandemic. This range of international projects is likely to offer an opportunity for further reflection, comparisons, dialogue and lessons in the future.

At the same time, we should not forget that despite the COVID-19 pandemic being, by definition, a global phenomenon, it has also been markedly culturally specific, local and hyper-local. Even in purely scientific terms, the identity of the virus itself has not been a global constant. Different strains and variants have emerged in different geographies and populations, and symptoms and morbidities have varied from country to country, creating very different patterns of disease across the world. Similarly, our responses to the pandemic and our standards of evidence and certainty – alongside modes of reasoning, ways of knowing and understanding – vary across cultural contexts, as we encounter different policymaking arrangements and civic communities. This is clear from the comparative work of the 'Lex Atlas' research in the *Pandemic and Beyond* portfolio, whose researchers examined dozens of countries' legal responses to the pandemic (King and Ferraz, 2021–23). Lessons learned in one country do not, therefore, translate cleanly to others.

Even within the UK, the response to COVID-19 was not uniformly governed or experienced. Nor did the disease spread evenly across the country. Time and time again, low-income households and communities, as well as groups with pre-existing vulnerabilities, felt the worst effects of both the disease and the measures put in place to protect the population. This pandemic was perhaps also one of the most challenging instances in which the arrangements for devolved administrations in Scotland, Wales and Northern Ireland, and the powers of the Westminster Government to oversee or coordinate national responses, were put to the test, prompting comparative analysis of the different modes and mechanisms of parliamentary review across the UK. This was complemented by scrutiny of data-driven approaches to decision-making and research that probed ethical and human rights issues. A deep delve into the situation in the UK provides us with valuable insight into the state of the nation – as well as our collective experience of the COVID-19 pandemic – in the early twenty-first century.

While arts and humanities research on COVID-19 in the UK is ongoing, and many are now engaged in the more considered process of retrospective analysis and critique, this series, produced at the endpoint of the rapid-response funding period, does represent a significant milestone. As such, it offers an opportunity to reflect on the multiple temporalities and intersectional crises that have characterised the first two years of the pandemic, along with the wider epistemic structures and infrastructures at stake in the delivery of this research portfolio. While COVID-19 had a fairly temporally precise beginning in the final days of 2019, at least as a distinct viral emergency, and was formalised as a global emergency with the World Health Organization's (WHO) declaration of a pandemic on 11 March 2020, it can also be understood as, at least in part, the product of a deeper crisis in terms of anthropogenic climate change and how we interact with the non-human (Gupta et al., 2021). COVID-19 has been a profoundly transformative, rupturing crisis, with over two million dead in Europe alone (WHO, 2022b). Worldwide, anxiety and depression increased by 25 per cent (WHO, 2022a), and access to professional services was challenging; over 100 million lost their jobs (WEF, 2021), and while some accessed furlough and insurance payments, freelancers and those in the gig economy were often ineligible (Fowler, 2020). COVID-19 identified and shone a light on 'key workers', who were defined as those whose work was deemed essential during the pandemic and who often turned out to be poorly paid, socially marginalised and previously 'invisible'. These workers included healthcare professionals as well as bus drivers, food retailers, refuse collectors and care home staff. While healthcare staff were routinely celebrated in the UK, most notably through the 'clap for our carers' phenomenon, this was not accompanied by material changes in stagnant pay or harmful working conditions, and others – such as domiciliary workers in care homes with older people – remained largely invisible.

As the virus began to transform the ways that we live and die, it pulled a series of overlapping crises and temporalities into tension, muddying any clean imagining of a shared pandemic trajectory. When the UK government announced extensive restrictions to movement and social life in the spring of 2020, disability scholars and activists noted that many disabled people had effectively been in 'lockdown' for years (Shakespeare et al., 2021). Likewise, COVID-19 intersected with deep-seated inequalities in race and health, landing disproportionately among people who had their ability to resist the virus eroded by generations of structural racism, and who were knowingly figured as disposable and exposed to greater risk than their white counterparts (Qureshi et al., 2022). Whole groups of people, including frail older people and those with underlying health conditions, were disproportionately negatively impacted. Other long and slow disasters and matters of justice (such as poverty, burnout in healthcare workers, or our inability to sufficiently care for the old) further altered the temporal bounds of the pandemic and fragmented our experiences of pandemic time (Baraitser and Salisbury, 2020). For doctors, nurses, cleaners and porters in overstretched hospital departments, time sped up (often in catastrophic ways); for those who were shielding or placed on furlough, the opposite was frequently true.

Among this profound and intractable messiness, attempts to impose a temporal order on the pandemic have always done a particular kind of political work. Across the conception and execution of these four volumes, rates of infection, illness and death have been in considerable flux; the state of the pandemic at the date of publication is impossible to know as we write this introduction in early 2023. We do know, however, that pandemics rarely – if ever – cleanly end (Greene and Vargha, 2020). The overlapping contexts and crises detailed above also frame wildly divergent apprehensions and realities of risk. Any intimation that we are becoming 'post-pandemic' must be met with a question the arts and humanities are uniquely poised to ask: for whom? The bereaved, still shielding, sufferers from 'long COVID', carers and healthcare professionals, after all, will continue to live pandemic time in different ways (Callard and Perego, 2021). One role of the arts and humanities amid this crisis is (or has been) to make and preserve *meaning* out of what has been experienced. In each of these volumes, 'rapid-response' arts and humanities work has had to navigate these slippery experiences of time. If many of our projects responded to the pandemic first in ways that were 'quick and dirty', acting to comprehend, forestall, or inform the present, the research assembled here is more inclined to the future, seeking to take a tentative and reflective step back from the immediacy of the pandemic while acknowledging its ongoing nature.

The format of the crisis-driven rapid-response call is itself an unusual approach to the organisation of arts and humanities research, with its distinctively longitudinal and reflective modes of relating to social problems. In one sense, this speedy deployment of the arts and humanities at a moment of crisis is welcome: it positions researchers within these disciplines as having skills that are critical for intervening in moments of emergency and lifts humanities research out of the epistemic position of providing commentary or representational analysis after the event. It thus refuses the disingenuous political position that cultural, literary, historical and theory-informed analysis is incompatible with the crisis resolution. Indeed, as this is a moment in which arts and humanities research is *itself* widely understood to be in crisis (see Thain et al., 2023), this instrumentalisation presents important new possibilities, and perhaps one or two pitfalls, for scholars within these disciplines. The assumption – implicit in the funding announcement – that research in the arts and humanities is already collaborative, engaged, pragmatic, problem-oriented, public-facing and interdisciplinary, an image which many in the humanities research community have been promoting for some years, often in the face of opposition from colleagues, is itself worthy of note.

This also follows a long-standing trend in which humanities research, whose structures have predominantly been based (somewhat stereotypically) on the model of a lone scholar, working diligently on their idiosyncratic topic over a period of years, is remade to resemble a more scientific model. Such a 'scientific model' notably involves the organisation of a project into research teams and work packages, the breaking down of disciplinary boundaries that are not methodologically salient, larger amounts of money being awarded to smaller numbers of research teams, the need to clearly articulate the public impact of research, and responsiveness to government and industry priorities. This trend has been clearly accelerated by the reorganisation of humanities research infrastructures during the COVID-19 pandemic, which, as we noted above, led to a much greater degree of collaboration, with several authors working remotely to write together, crossing institutional, geographical, disciplinary and hierarchical boundaries. The epistemic effects of such reorganisation have been real – and mixed. The organisation of research, after all, plays a large role in governing not just the type of writing possible in such circumstances, but also what research can and cannot be done. While the funding that framed the *Pandemic and Beyond* portfolio opened up many new possibilities for humanities researchers, it simultaneously foreclosed others. Scholars without a desire to work in teams, whose research did not need significant money or have clearly defined short- to medium-term impacts, will have struggled to contribute; a significant loss that mostly remains invisible. This portfolio showcases many new opportunities, but it also hides the opportunity costs – not only for humanities work directly on COVID-19, but for humanities research generally, as already scarce resources were poured into immediate responses to a single public health crisis.

In the context of a UK government research funding strategy which, as the March 2023 HEPI report notes, 'appears to downplay the position of the Arts and Humanities in the UK's ambition to become a "science superpower"' (Thain et al., 2023: 19), there is a wider political dimension to this, too. The COVID-19 crisis also coincided with a series of crises around Brexit, one of the most prominent of which concerned the possibility of the UK's participation in (or exclusion from) the EU's Horizon research programme. This created a context in which research was wielded openly as a token of national competitiveness, and international collaboration was reframed as a luxury that could be removed at a government's whim. While the UK focus of the *Pandemic and Beyond* research shielded this portfolio from some of these pressures, we nevertheless continuously faced the need to demonstrate, in a political climate ill-disposed to critical humanities thinking, the relevance, success, impact or transformational potential of this body of research. Against this backdrop, it was often tempting to frame our work to make it align with (party) political slogans such as 'build back better' or 'levelling up' to demonstrate a willingness to engage with political priorities. The need to establish such 'synergies' is now a common and perhaps unavoidable feature of research coordination and curation efforts such as that of *Pandemic and Beyond*. Indeed, the research we share through these volumes should also be understood in the context of a wider, global attack on the humanities, whether departmental closures in the United Kingdom, the driver for teaching efficiencies in Denmark, or legislative attacks in countries such as Hungary and the United States. The quick pivot to rapid-response work on COVID-19 is both an affirmative rebuttal to such attacks (our work is indeed both important and useful) *and* a frank recognition of how successful they have been (our work is only viable to the extent that we can successfully position it as both important and useful). Our work, then, while bearing witness to the importance, usefulness and practical applicability of arts and humanities research in crisis contexts, also situates itself within broader national and international debates about the role arts and humanities play in fostering and sustaining the creative and open-ended critical thinking that underpins democratic political structures.

The *Pandemic and Beyond* series

The aim of this series is to preserve the breadth of the approaches taken by *Pandemic and Beyond* researchers in addressing the crisis, showcasing a form of arts and humanities research that has learned how to respond to, and mitigate, COVID-19 as it unfolded, and that has constantly adapted its methods and research questions to ongoing developments and the needs of research participants. Reflecting the variety of the *Pandemic and Beyond* research portfolio, the chapters we have selected range from in-depth reflection on schools of thought and social and governance structures that have influenced approaches to the pandemic to those that are much more 'hands-on'. These latter chapters address subjects sometimes sidelined in conventional academic writing, as their focus on working structures, industrial practices and lived experience does not always lend itself easily to conceptual debates and theorisation.

Written from the retrospective vantage point of late 2022 and the first months of 2023, these chapters offer a rare insight into the findings and often invisible facets of research projects whose primary focus was rapid on-the-ground impact, knowledge exchange, and direct engagement with communities, organisations and decision-makers. The chapters we collect not only offer reflection on what the research teams achieved, but also on what could be learned from their experiences to guide future responses to ongoing, accelerating and emerging crises, whether in relation to climate, migration, violent conflict, the threat of vaccine-resistant coronavirus variants, or other pathogens that could develop into new pandemics. The result is a series which models how, in responding to a crisis, the creativity, cultural sensitivity, community-reach and knowledge base of arts and humanities researchers can be one of the best tools to understand a novel virus in all its dimensions, steer policy and alleviate suffering on the ground.

In our volume *Adaptation and Resilience in the Performing Arts*, we explore how live performing arts in the UK innovated during public health restrictions to everyday life to overcome the obstacles to co-presence and performance in shared spaces that were a side-effect of pandemic mitigation measures. The volume explores the financial hardship and mental health impacts experienced by industry professionals as governmental discourses regarding the 'viability' of arts careers, alongside the difficulties of connecting with networks and accessing arts opportunities, put a particular strain on creative workers and freelancers in the UK at a time when some Latin American countries were leading the way in valuing and supporting the arts. Against this backdrop of existential struggle for creative workers, this volume celebrates the ingenuity and creativity of artists and researchers who applied themselves to finding both digital and analogue solutions to the problem of co-presence, and who, in so doing, broadened the access of previously marginalised communities to live performing arts. It highlights projects that explored how motion-capture and green screen technologies can enable performers to come together despite geographical distance and interact in a shared virtual space to create new work, and how such digital work affects their art, wellbeing and ability to reach wider audiences. It also champions the value of local initiatives in outdoor spaces and suggests avenues for artists and local governments to reimagine towns and cities as performance venues in which diverse communities can gather to celebrate their location and ability to communally enjoy art amid a pandemic.

The mobilisation of existing natural, community and cultural assets and resources to support individual and community wellbeing – conducted at speed and often using novel modes of delivery – was a notable feature of pandemic responses across the UK. Our volume *Creative Approaches to Wellbeing* presents detailed examples of research looking at how these kinds of activities sought to address issues such as the challenges of isolation, to support health and care workers, or to create spaces that could enable coping, recovery or renewal. Common to the chapters here are reflections on what it means and what tools and systems might be needed if we are to develop resilience during and after such crises in future, alongside examination of ideas of 'vulnerability'. Authors bring to these discussions a particular focus on the experiences of those most marginalised during the pandemic because of mental or physical ill-health, age, or due to deep-seated structural and systemic inequalities. Individual contributions include an interrogation of the idea of 'togetherness' itself; an invitation to consider the benefits of 'walking creatively', a study of the work of small organisations in promoting health through interaction with urban nature; and investigations of the contributions of the cultural, museum and literary heritage sectors to wellbeing. Looking forward, authors invite us to consider how adaptations to ways of working for individuals, within organisations, and even at the level of a whole city region, could lead to changes in provision and lessons for practice.

Knowing COVID-19 looks at how different kinds of knowledge and meaning have been created and communicated, and the repercussions this has had – and continues to have – for how COVID-19 is managed, experienced, understood and remembered. Knowledge-making, it suggests, took various forms, and these are reflected in the diversity of chapters this volume curates. In the first instance, it demonstrates a rich humanities tradition of constructive critique, as 'official' communications around 'staying home', 'keeping distance', safety on buses, lateral flow testing, and vaccine hesitancy are tested and interrogated. Through this collective work, we see one of the clear, indisputable values of the humanities; their attentiveness to the human, and the clarifying or reflective power this might have had with greater embeddedness in policy and information design. In the second instance – and frequently both are accomplished in the same short chapter – this volume collects a series of interventions which set out specifically to create and sustain meaning, particularly when dominant cultural narratives over the pandemic rely on those meanings slipping away from political or popular memory. Thus, we have rich and detailed explorations of the experiences of museum workers, people told to 'stay home', older victims of gender-based violence, people with deafblindness, and racialised nurses working in the NHS; as well as extensive reflection on what it was like to make the projects which formalised this knowledge work. Taken as a whole, this volume critiques and redefines pandemic epistemologies, assembling a partial blueprint for making future crises legible.

Finally, *Governance, Democracy and Ethics in Crisis-Decision-Making* explores what it means to be in a situation in which rational or epistemic framings of the COVID-19 pandemic, with a focus on data and scientific ways of knowing the world, rub up against more entangled accounts. In these accounts, humans, the virus and governance arrangements coexist as a broader, relational whole. Human connections, personal fulfilment and social groupings are inextricably intertwined with matters (and meanings) of governance, ethics and authority, the rule of law, the economy and, crucially, public health. Looking at issues ranging from the authority of the WHO and the power of data during an emergency, to the role of public engagement as a source of policy evidence, we reflect on what it means to govern *ethically* in a pandemic, and whether the expected standards and norms of public life, evidence and decision-making should be different in times of crisis. We also reflect on how the long tail of the pandemic seems impossible to disentangle from a reduced trust in power and authority, creating an urgent need for ethics to move beyond normative assertions of the law and regulations. Our authors provide some suggestions as to how these things might be balanced more ethically and effectively in the future.

In 2020 and 2021, when televised government briefings on COVID-19 remained commonplace, ministers insisted time and again that they were 'following the science' (Colman et al., 2021). Even when critics called the accuracy of this rhetorical device into question, they rarely troubled the governing logic that, were we only willing to follow it, scientific and medical evidence offered an unclouded route map through the pandemic. However, '[c]oping with the pandemic was (for the lucky majority who were not severely ill) not so much a medical crisis as an existential one' (Thain et al., 2023: 13); indeed, given the complex interplay of social, cultural, ethical, economic and political framings of health, illness and disease, there is no such thing as a purely medical crisis (Ryan, 2022). The *Pandemic and Beyond* series reveals how the arts and humanities research community rose to the challenge of this complexity, growing in confidence as it became increasingly clear that our methodologies, forms of knowledge and creative mindsets were key not only to tackling this all-encompassing human emergency, but, in so doing, to alleviating human suffering. As one of our researchers commented:

> What has been evident across our COVID-19 research projects is that arts-based research methods and approaches can generate much more nuanced narratives, capture the complex experiences and engage people that wouldn't otherwise find research accessible. Whilst of course medical research in such a crisis is fundamental, so too is understanding different people's experiences, responses and how their lives have been impacted so we can make more effective policies and support people's recovery and resilience looking forward. (Aebischer et al., 2022: 30)

If, as another *Pandemic and Beyond* researcher put it, this work 'has been a game-changer' in revealing the skill and generosity of the research community (Aebischer et al., 2022: 29), then it is also a call to action in the future, as we face a multitude of ongoing and emerging crises, from climate to migration and economic decline, which demand collective and civic responsibility and the willingness to continue to combine nuanced and context-sensitive thinking with a solutions-focused approach.

Without the vast collective knowledge, experience, methodological tools and expertise on which this type of research draws, our responses to ongoing challenges and future crises can only ever be impoverished. Expecting politicians of the future to say that they are 'following the humanities' might be wishful thinking. A pandemic response which made more extensive use of the kinds of evidence and interventions on show in these volumes, however, would have been far more attentive to questions of power and justice; understood how, why and when particular people felt – and became – less safe; had a far better handle on how we engage with public health advice or vaccination drives; and begun from a richer knowledge of what the arts can do to keep us feeling human in the most difficult of circumstances. As a recent essay on climate change suggests, the arts and humanities have to be equal to the series of interlocking emergencies which frame our present historical moment (Pietsch and Flanagan, 2020). Over the past three years, scholars and practitioners have painstakingly built a 'pandemic humanities' – and a pandemic arts and cultural sector – which demonstrates that the arts and humanities are more than equal to the task. Creating the conditions for this work to (continue to) thrive must, surely, constitute one of the best forms of crisis preparedness we have.

Notes

1 Funded by UKRI/AHRC from February 2021 to February 2022, grant reference AH/W000881/1. The project's legacy website is housed at https://pandemicandbeyond.exeter.ac.uk/ and will be maintained until February 2028.
2 *The Pandemic and Beyond* was responsible specifically for the AHRC segment of the research portfolio created by the UKRI call, first published on 31 March 2020, for 'ideas that address COVID-19'. A version of the call updated on 21 September 2020 is available at www.ukri.org/opportunity/get-funding-for-ideas-that-address-covid-19/ (last accessed 4 February 2023).
3 For a map of projects focusing on COVID-19 funded by UKRI, see https://strategicfutures.org/TopicMaps/UKRI/research_map.html (last accessed 4 February 2023).

References

Aebischer, Pascale, *et al.* (2022), *The Pandemic and Beyond: The Arts and Humanities Contribution to Covid Research and Recovery*. Final Project Report. Available at: http://hdl.handle.net/10871/132640 (accessed 30 March 2023).

Baraitser, Lisa and Laura Salisbury (2020), 'Containment, delay, mitigation': Waiting and care in the time of a pandemic [version 2; peer review: 2 approved]. *Wellcome Open Res* 5, 129. DOI: 10.12688/wellcomeopenres.15970.2

Callard, Felicity and Elisa Perego (2021), How and why patients made Long Covid. *Social Science & Medicine* 268, 113426. DOI: 10.1016/j.socscimed.2020.113426

Colman, Elien, *et al.* (2021), Following the science? Views from scientists on government advisory boards during the COVID-19 pandemic: A qualitative interview study in five European Countries. *BMJ Global Health* 6, e006928. DOI: 10.1136/bmjgh-2021-006928

Fowler, Damian (28 March 2020), Unemployment during coronavirus: The psychology of job loss. BBC Worklife. Available at: www.bbc.com/worklife/article/20200327-unemployment-during-coronavirus-the-psychology-of-job-loss (accessed 30 February 2023).

Greene, Jeremy A. and Dora Vargha (2020), How epidemics end. *Boston Review*, 30 June. Available at: www.bostonreview.net/articles/jeremy-greene-dora-vargha-how-epidemics-end-or-dont/ (accessed 30 March 2023).

Gupta, Saloni, Barry T. Rouse and Pranita P. Sarangi (2021), Did climate change influence the emergence, transmission, and expression of the COVID-19 pandemic? *Frontiers in Medicine* 8, 769208. DOI: 10.3389/fmed.2021.769208

King, Jeff and Octávio Ferraz (eds) (2021–23), *The Oxford Compendium of National Legal Responses to COVID-19*. Oxford: Oxford Constitutional Law, https://oxcon.ouplaw.com/home/OCC19. Last accessed 4 February 2023.

Pietsch, Tamson and Frances Flanagan (2020), Here we stand: Temporal thinking in urgent times. *History Australia* 17.2, 252–271. DOI: 10.1080/14490854.2020.1758577

Pirgova-Morgan, Luba (2022), Exploring the impact of COVID-19 on GCRF and Newton Projects: A research report by PRAXIS: Arts and Humanities for Global Development. Leeds: University of Leeds, PRAXIS: Arts and Humanities for Global Development 2022. Available at: https://changingthestory.leeds.ac.uk/wp-content/uploads/sites/178/2022/06/University-of-Leeds-PRAXIS-COVID-19-Report-Final-Single-0422.pdf (accessed 30 March 2023).

Qureshi, Irtiza, *et al.* (2022), Healthcare workers from diverse ethnicities and their perceptions of risk and experiences of risk management during the COVID-19 pandemic: Qualitative insights from the United Kingdom-REACH Study. *Frontiers in Medicine* 9, 930904. DOI: 10.3389/fmed.2022.930904

Ryan, J. Michael (2022), Coda: Global consciousness of COVID-19: Where can we go from here? In Irene Gammel and Jason Wang (eds), *Creative Resilience and COVID-19: Figuring the Everyday in a Pandemic*. Abingdon: Routledge, pp. 195–200.

Shakespeare, Tom, Florence Ndagire and Queen E. Seketi (2021), Triple jeopardy: Disabled people and the COVID-19 pandemic. *The Lancet* 397.10282, 1331–1333. DOI: 10.1016/S0140–6736(21)00625–5

Thain, Marion, *et al.* (2023), The humanities in the UK today: What's going on? *HEPI Report* 159, March. Available at: www.hepi.ac.uk/wp-content/uploads/2023/03/The-Humanities-in-the-UK-Today-Whats-Going-On.pdf (accessed 30 March 2023).

WEF (2021), Covid employment global job loss. World Economic Forum, 4 February. Available at: www.weforum.org/agenda/2021/02/covid-employment-global-job-loss/ (accessed 20 February 2023).

WHO (2 March 2022a), COVID-19 pandemic triggers 25% increase in prevalence of anxiety and depression worldwide. WHO News Release. Available at: www.who.int/news/item/02–03–2022-covid-19-pandemic-triggers-25-increase-in-prevalence-of-anxiety-and-depression-worldwide (accessed 20 February 2023).

WHO (12 May 2022b), Two million confirmed deaths from COVID-19 in the European region. WHO News Release. Available at: www.who.int/europe/news/item/12–05-2022-two-million-confirmed-deaths-from-covid-19-in-the-european-region (accessed 20 February 2023).

Figures

Unless otherwise stated, all rights are reserved. For permission to reproduce any of these images please contact the rightsholder.

1.1	Still from *Use Your Head to Stop the Spread* (short video), part of the 'You're Never Alone on the Bus' series (© 2021 Joseph Turp and Routes to Safety)	24
2.1	Still from VR video (Altered Perception Exhibition, 2022): Issy in her kitchen arranging flowers	41
3.1	Laboratory testing versus point-of-care testing	62
3.2	COVID-19 self-test	64
3.3	Overview of techniques to enable decision-making in the design process (Walker et al., 2022)	67
3.4	Different versions to indicate the action 'rotate the swab'	69
3.5	Examples B and C show versions of 'rotate the swab' using a ghosted shape	69
3.6	Different versions to indicate 'squeeze the tube'	70
3.7	Different versions of the actions 'rotate the swab' and 'remove the swab while squeezing the tube' showing the actions with no hand, one or two hands	70
3.8	Prototype point-of-use instructions for COVID-19 lateral flow tests, developed using evidence from the research project and established knowledge in the design of instructional texts	72

3.9	Application of the approach to an SOP (Standard Operating Procedure) to operate a lateral flow test for influenza	74
3.10	SOP Quick Guide, with edited text and illustrations to include the key elements	75
3.11	Internal Quality Control (IQC), using the same conventions, including horizontal bands to separate the component parts. To distinguish it from the SOP and Quick Guide, a different colour is used for the key steps	76
3.12	Pages of the toolkit 'User-friendly point-of-use instructions for home use diagnostic tests: guidance and tools'. Each page in the toolkit summarises key issues and provides captioned or annotated illustrations to explain the key points	80
4.1	Map by Niccolo	97
4.2	Map by Aurelius	98

Contributors

Pascale Aebischer is Professor of Shakespeare and Early Modern Performance Studies at the University of Exeter. She is a specialist in performance technologies who, during the COVID-19 pandemic, worked on Digital Theatre Transformation (AHRC) and took on the leadership of an interdisciplinary team at the University of Exeter for The Pandemic and Beyond: The Arts and Humanities Contribution to Covid Research and Recovery (AHRC-funded project). Building on this work, she is now Co-Lead, with Karen Gray (University of Bristol), of the British Academy-funded Pandemic Preparedness in the Live Performing Arts: Lessons to Learn from COVID-19 project (2023–2024).

Alison Blunt is Professor of Geography at Queen Mary University of London, Co-Director of the Centre for Studies of Home (a partnership between Queen Mary and the Museum of the Home) and was Principal Investigator on the Arts and Humanities Research Council-funded project Stay Home Stories. Her recent publications include, with Robyn Dowling, *Home* (Routledge, 2022, 2nd edition).

Josefina Bravo, PhD, is a practising information designer and Lecturer at the University of Reading, UK. In her practice and research, she has focused on the design of user-friendly health information, emergency information and education materials. She is particularly interested in user instructions and the range of visual techniques that can be used to enable comprehension of instructional text.

Kathy Burrell is Professor of Migration Geographies at the University of Liverpool, UK, and was a Co-Investigator on the Arts and Humanities Research Council-funded project Stay Home Stories. She is currently working on a British Academy-funded project on Polish experiences of the post-Brexit Settled Status regime, as well as researching the UK's refugee hosting programme Homes for Ukraine.

Fred Cooper is a historian of loneliness and shame, presently working at the University of Bristol as a Senior Research Associate on the Wellcome-funded Epistemic Injustice in Health Care project (EPIC). With Luna Dolezal and Arthur Rose, he co-authored *Covid-19 and Shame: Political Emotions and Public Health in the UK* (Bloomsbury Academic, 2023), and was Co-Investigator on the AHRC-funded project, Scenes of Shame and Stigma in COVID-19.

Elizabeth Crooke is Professor of Heritage and Museum Studies at Ulster University, UK, and Principal Investigator of the UKRI-funded project Museums, Crisis and Covid19: Vitality and Vulnerabilities. Her research focuses on what museums bring to society and how we engage with them.

Luna Dolezal is Professor of Philosophy and Medical Humanities at the University of Exeter, UK. She is Principal Investigator of the Shame and Medicine Project (2020–2025), funded by the Wellcome Trust. She collaborated with Arthur Rose and Fred Cooper on the Scenes of Shame and Stigma in COVID-19 project (2020–2022), funded by the AHRC, and they co-authored the book *Covid-19 and Shame: Political Emotions and Public Health in the UK* (Bloomsbury Academic, 2023).

Alexander Edwards has a background in fundamental immunology combined with expertise in biochemical engineering. He is an interdisciplinary researcher focused on solving current and future healthcare challenges by combining the latest biology, biochemistry, chemistry and physics. Working at the interface between academic technology discovery and industrial development, he has experience of both fundamental science and the commercialisation of new technology, especially in the area of clinical diagnostic.

Azadeh Emadi is a Senior Lecturer and video maker at the University of Glasgow, UK (Film and TV Department). Her scholarly and creative work intends to address socio-environmental issues and create space for cultural dialogues by investigating digital materiality and perception, visual aesthetics, alternative approaches to image making and technologies of perception.

Georgina Endfield is Professor of Environmental History and Associate Pro Vice Chancellor for the Research Environment and Postgraduate Research at the University of Liverpool, UK. She was Co-Investigator on the Arts and Humanities Research Council-funded project Stay Home Stories and is currently working on a book on societal relationships with the weather through time in a UK context.

David Farrell-Banks is a Practitioner Research Associate at the Fitzwilliam Museum, University of Cambridge, UK. His work explores the personal, political and affective role of the past on present-day lived experience.

Ken Fero, PhD, is Assistant Professor at the Research Centre for Global Education at Coventry University, UK, as well as the Director of Migrant Media, a radical documentary film collective working on issues of race, class and resistance.

Des Fitzgerald is Professor of Medical Humanities and Social Sciences in the Radical Humanities Laboratory, University College Cork, Ireland. His most recent book is *The City of Today Is a Dying Thing* (Faber and Faber, 2024).

Karen Gray is a researcher with a particular interest in work at the intersection between culture, health and wellbeing. She is currently Senior Research Associate at the School for Policy Studies at the University of Bristol. During the pandemic she worked on the Impacts of COVID-19 on the UK Cultural Sector (AHRC) project with the Centre for Cultural Value, as well as The Pandemic and Beyond: The Arts and Humanities Contribution to Covid Research and Recovery (AHRC-funded). In 2023–2024 she built on this experience, co-leading with Pascale Aebischer the British

Academy-funded project Pandemic Preparedness in the Live Performing Arts: Lessons to Learn from COVID-19.

Amanda Holt is Professor of Criminology at the University of Roehampton, London, UK. Her research work focuses on families, young people and harm and she has published widely on topics concerned with parenting and youth justice, family violence and homicide and research methodologies. Her books include *Adolescent-to-Parent Abuse: Current Understandings in Research, Policy and Practice* (Policy Press, 2013) and the edited collection *Working with Adolescent Violence and Abuse towards Parents: Approaches and Contexts for Intervention* (Routledge, 2016). She is a Trustee of Family Lives, the national family support charity.

Paul Hurley is an artist-researcher working inside and outside of universities. He specialises in creating qualitative, participatory and artistic research and engagement projects, and is interested in exploring human–non-human entanglements, whether they are microbes, laboratory animals or postnature wildlife. While Paul's roots are in the fields of Performance and Participatory Art and More-than-Human Geographies, he is currently working with the Centre for Higher Education Practice at the University of Southampton, UK, creating programmes in researcher development.

Miri Lawrence is a Rabbi and researcher. She was a Postdoctoral Researcher on the Arts and Humanities Research Council-funded project Stay Home Stories, and Curator of Liberal Judaism's Lily's Legacy Project.

Jess Moriarty is Principal Lecturer in Creative Writing at the University of Brighton, UK, and Co-Director of its Centre for Arts and Wellbeing. She is course leader for the Creative Writing BA, English Language and Creative Writing BA, English Literature and Creative Writing BA and for the Creative Writing MA. Jess's research focuses on autoethnography, community engagement and pedagogy in writing practice. She has published extensively on creative writing pedagogy, autoethnography and community engagement. Her current book (with Christina Reading), *Walking for Creative*

Recovery (Triarchy Press, 2022) adopts an autoethnographic approach and explores creative practice as a method for supporting wellbeing.

Lesley Murray is Professor in Spatial Sociology at the University of Brighton, UK, where her research centres on urban mobilities. Lesley has published extensively in the field of mobilities; topics include the intersections between mobile and visual methods and gendered mobilities, children's mobilities. She has co-authored a book on *Children's Mobilities* (Palgrave Macmillan, 2019) and co-edited five transdisciplinary collections: *Mobile Methodologies* (Palgrave Macmillan, 2010); *Researching and Representing Mobilities* (Palgrave Macmillan, 2014); *Intergenerational Mobilities* (Routledge, 2016); *Families in Motion* (Emerald Publishing, 2019); and *Sensory Transformations* (Routledge, 2023).

Eithne Nightingale is a writer, film maker and researcher. She was a Postdoctoral Researcher on the Arts and Humanities Research Council-funded project Stay Home Stories and directed the related podcasts and films. Her book *Child Migrant Voices in Modern Britain: Oral Histories from 1930s to the Present Day* (Bloomsbury, 2024) was based on her PhD research on child migration undertaken at Queen Mary University of London.

Alastair Owens is Professor of Historical Geography at Queen Mary University of London and was a Co-Investigator on the Arts and Humanities Research Council-funded project Stay Home Stories. He is currently working on a book about the response of Church of England clergy living and working in urban parishes to the so-called 'crisis' of the British inner city in the late twentieth century

Anandi Ramamurthy is Professor of Media and Culture at Sheffield Hallam University, UK. Her research explores questions of race and representation in British and global cultures using an interdisciplinary approach. She was the Principal Investigator for the UKRI/AHRC- funded project Nursing Narratives: Racism and the Pandemic. Her previous books include *Imperial Persuaders: Images of Africa and Asia in British Advertising* (Manchester University

Press, 2003); *Black Star: Britain's Asian Youth Movements* (Pluto Press, 2013); *Struggling to Be Seen: The Travails of Palestinian Cinema* (Daraja, 2020; with Paul Kelemen).

Caroline Redhead is a Research Fellow in the Centre for Social Ethics and Policy, part of the Law Department at the University of Manchester. Having worked as a commercial solicitor for many years, in the UK and in Hong Kong, she moved from private practice to academia in 2020. Her research interests lie broadly in the dynamic interplay between law, ethics (particularly bioethics) and social change.

Emma Roe is a transdisciplinary scholar and Professor of More-than-Human Geographies in the School of Geography and Environment at the University of Southampton, UK. Current research addresses steps towards a net zero agro-food system; tackling the rise in anti-microbial resistance and other microbial risks in and beyond the food system; and laboratory animal care, breeding and supply practices. Emma is often found working with those outside her discipline and with community and industry partners. She is the co-author of *Food and Animal Welfare* (Bloomsbury, 2018), and co-editor of *Participatory Research in More-than-Human Worlds* (Routledge, 2018) and *Researching Animal Research* (Manchester University Press, 2023).

Arthur Rose is a Senior Research Fellow at the University of Exeter, UK, where he contributes to the Shame and Medicine Project, funded by the Wellcome Trust. Together with Fred Cooper and Luna Dolezal, he worked on the AHRC-funded project Scenes of Shame and Stigma in COVID-19 (2020–2022), for which they co-authored the book *Covid-19 and Shame: Political Emotions and Public Health in the UK* (Bloomsbury Academic, 2023).

Melanie Smallman is Associate Professor in Science and Technology Studies and Co-Director of the Responsible Research and Innovation Hub at University College London (UCL). Melanie's research looks at the role of science and innovation (particularly data-technologies and artificial intelligence [AI]) in increasing inequality, and how the social impacts of these technologies can be included in ethical and policy considerations.

Victoria Tischler is Professor of Behavioural Science in the Faculty of Health and Medical Sciences at the University of Surrey, UK. She is a Chartered Psychologist and Associate Fellow of the British Psychological Society. Her research focuses on creativity and mental health and multisensory (especially olfactory) approaches to promoting healthy ageing. She has expertise in medical and health humanities and on untrained (outsider) art.

Charlotte Veal, PhD, is a Lecturer in Landscape in the School of Architecture, Planning and Landscape and Co-Director of The Landscape Collaboratory at Newcastle University, UK. She has an accelerating international research profile for interdisciplinary research at the intersection of bodies, performance and (bio-)security. Her research into interspecies relations (virus, seaweed) is underpinned by post-humanist and post-structuralist thinking in conjunction with experimental creative-arts methods with transdisciplinary audiences.

Jacky Waldock is Faculty Impact Fellow and Deputy Director of the Centre for Arts, Society and the Environment at the University of Liverpool, UK. She was previously a Postdoctoral Researcher on the Arts and Humanities Research Council-funded project Stay Home Stories. She is a specialist in sonic studies, researching sonic place-making and listening cultures in the home and has published a number of essays and articles on these topics.

Sue Walker is Professor of Typography at the University of Reading, UK. She has a longstanding interest in the history, theory and practice of information design. Her current research involves interdisciplinary working in communication design for antimicrobial resistance and in adolescent mental health, science communication for young people and COVID-19 rapid-response projects on home-testing.

Annabelle Wilkins is a Postdoctoral Researcher on the Nordforsk-funded Making It Home project at Kingston University London, and was a Postdoctoral Researcher on the Arts and Humanities Research Council-funded project Stay Home Stories. She is the author of *Migration, Work and Home-Making in the City: Dwelling and Belonging among Vietnamese Communities in London* (Routledge, 2019).

Sandra Wilks is Associate Professor at the University of Southampton, UK, with more than 20 years' experience in the field of applied biofilm research, including highly interdisciplinary projects on food protection and medical device use and design. She has a particular interest in understanding the complexity of microbial communities, how to detect low levels of pathogens, and how we can communicate and gain a better understanding of microbial risk.

Introduction – Knowing COVID-19: The pandemic and beyond

Fred Cooper and Des Fitzgerald

In April 2021, the UK Government announced that free lateral flow tests (LFTs) for COVID-19 were to be made available to the public through pharmacies and test centres, following several months of trials in schools and universities. The announcement came on the heel of a growing realisation, through the first year of the COVID-19 pandemic, that large numbers of people with the virus experienced no symptoms at all, or mild symptoms that could be difficult to discern from seasonal influenza or the common cold. This posed a problem during a period when, in many countries, pandemic governance was still operating through a strategy of isolation and containment, at least formally: without regular mass testing, significant numbers of people would continue to avoid quarantine or self-isolation, and thus spread infection. LFTs – cheaper, quicker and easier to use than the more reliable polymerase chain reaction (PCR) tests used at official testing sites – were a plausible part of the answer. Additionally, in a comparative international context where poor pandemic planning and a series of government omissions and miscalculations had resulted in high rates of infection and death, a mass testing programme framed by hyperbolic rhetoric was a means for the UK Government to save face (Cooper et al., 2023). Indeed, as some pointed out at the time, the relatively high number of false negative results may well have made the tests very possibly inappropriate for home use – leading to a conclusion that what was at stake was much more political posturing than any concerted attempt at pandemic management (see Bunn, 2021).

LFTs went on to become one of the truly iconic technologies of the pandemic. In many places, people became wearyingly familiar with the small rectangular bars of mostly white, and vaguely clinical, plastic, dipped in the middle to provide visual access to a results strip. This strip, in turn, was usually marked with a letter C (for control) about a third of the way down, and a T (for test) a further third of the way down. There was a pencil-tip-sized hole for the user's saliva at one end, and a (frequently disregarded) identifying number or barcode to report the result on the other. Despite multiple manufacturers and different waves of distribution, these essentials never changed much. During peaks of infection over subsequent months, social media users' feeds were often overtaken by friends' and acquaintances' images of their just-used LFTs. One red line (at C) usually produced something like wry relief, uncertainty (given the unreliability of the tests) or even joy; while the dreaded second T line, denoting a positive result, often led to a shared sense of anxiety or concern – for some, indeed, a deep and justified fear – but also, sometimes, a dark humour too.

The lateral flow test, we can say now with some perspective, has been one of the major sources through which the pandemic became quite literally *known* to many people, at both individual and collective scales. It was a cheap, mass-produced, visually oriented medical device; a product through which the presence (or absence) of COVID-19 became briefly legible to a population mostly with no clinical or diagnostic training. Indeed, between the saliva-hole and the thin red line(s), the test became something like what is known in Science and Technology Studies (following Bruno Latour) as a black box – an artefact in which a whole range of social and technical controversies are neatly packed away and rendered invisible. The red lines denoting the result were all that came to matter – both technically and politically (see Latour, 1987). Indeed, the visual charisma of the LFT's signalling system (the red lines blooming and fading; sometimes appearing and disappearing as infection waxes and wanes) trades quite explicitly on this shifting, contingent relationship between what may or may not be knowable, as well as what we may be called upon to do (as both epidemiological and political actors) in the wake of that knowledge.

There is, of course, an extensive literature on the production of visual technology in science and medicine, as cinematic techniques, screen-based media, medical devices and subsequent forms of data visualisation came together to make the body and its pathologies knowable (see e.g. Cartwright, 1995; Halpern, 2014). As Lisa

Cartwright among others has convincingly shown, representations of the body are now deeply entwined in the visual culture of the life sciences, as well as the very different technologies that make this culture possible. We might well analyse the LFT through this history and take it as a point from which to make sense of the visual culture of public health in a pandemic era. We might think carefully through questions of usability, shape, legibility, display and communication, to attach this performatively banal and clinical object, with its sad little paper-strip heart, to a wider literature on biomedicine's investment in visual reason. This would, of course, be a worthwhile project – and one, indeed, likely underway somewhere as we write.

And yet, as Sue Walker, Josefina Bravo and Al Edwards make clear in their contribution to this volume (Chapter 3), these questions of the knowable and the legible, as they were embodied quite precisely in the LFT, were not at all confined to researchers in the medical or life sciences. Or, to put it otherwise: to the extent that the LFT is what the historian Hans-Jörg Rheinberger (1997) calls an epistemic thing, a site of unknowability within a carefully constructed technical apparatus, then the people constructing that apparatus are not only people with engineering and diagnostic expertise. There are also people with deep expertise in information and communication design; in what we know about the visual organisation of text; in research on how best to illustrate the action designated by an instruction like 'rotate'. There are people with expertise in the history and sociology of how colours work across and between cultures; in how you know whether people actually followed (or didn't follow) an instruction in practice; in the multiple ways that bureaucratic and legal hurdles might constrain how a product could be narrated; and in the basic methodological questions of how to run a successful stakeholder workshop. Which is to say that a great deal of the technical expertise that makes the test possible is expertise that we would usually associate with 'the humanities' (or perhaps with the humanities and social sciences). If we are to understand the sites of technical expertise that are holding the LFT together as a diagnostic object, if we open up the black box, as Latour has it, then we will quickly find ourselves out of the laboratory and the engineering workshop, and instead in the design studio, in the participant workshop, talking to the artist, ringing the anthropologist, checking with the lawyer, or trying to find a translator. What we very quickly realise – what, indeed, *was* realised, in the early stages of the pandemic – is that if we want to know how well a scientific apparatus works, we don't only need to know how reliably a red line at 'T' signals a true result. We need to know how real human beings – in their kitchens, surrounded by empty cereal bowls and children's toys, under pressure to go into work, not at all used to administering their own diagnostic tests, perhaps confused and a little irritated, and likely not feeling so great – are actually going to interpret, make sense of and render knowable the lines (or lack of them) on the strip.

This relationship between humanities research and knowledge is what draws the chapters in this volume together. The authors below (and the projects they discuss) are united by a shared commitment to making the COVID-19 pandemic knowable. But they enact this commitment not in a secondary or reactive sense – for example, in historical or sociological reflection on how epidemiology or the life sciences produced knowledge of COVID – but in the primary sense of figuring out how humanities expertise can be a part of producing new knowledge on a novel infectious disease. Each chapter in this volume reports from a project that brought this expertise to bear on one or more knotty questions of what we knew or didn't know about COVID-19 and its impact: whether this was how to communicate risks on public transport; how deafblind people were going to navigate a world without touch; how racism in the health service was likely to impact on differential exposure to illness and disease; or how people would bear, experientially, a sudden injunction to 'stay home'. Most particularly, in the context of an official pandemic response which was frequently characterised by an inattention to, sometimes a knowing neglect of, pressing questions of complexity and justice, scholars in a number of different disciplinary contexts initiated programmes of work which set out explicitly to compensate for these epistemic, practical and ethical shortcomings. Humanities researchers, far from a relationship with crisis characterised by temporally removed attempts to make meaning, or by oblique and slow pathways to impact, have been right in the thick of things, bringing their expertise and training to bear on some of the most critical epistemic and *technical* questions at the heart of the pandemic. In the case of the lateral flow test – but also far more broadly – humanities research ceases to be a set of stories about meaning and experience; it is rather a set of critical, technical and rigorous procedures through which we come to know what is happening to our bodies, precisely at the moment of crisis, and according to which we might begin to take reparative (or other) action.

This transformation implies some important consequences, both for how we think about an infectious disease pandemic and how we think about the humanities. First, although COVID has been mediatised since its emergence almost exclusively as a clinical and scientific problem – think of sombre announcements by political figures flanked by senior medics, perhaps with that now over-familiar red and grey pinhead characterisation of the SARS-CoV-2 virus hovering somewhere in the background – it is now clear that this framing fundamentally misunderstood both the disease and the pandemic we would come to know. Even at the very moment of emergence, which was marked by outbreaks of anti-Chinese racism and violence in multiple places, as well as a consumer rush for scarce goods like hand sanitiser and toilet rolls, it was clear that knowing COVID – as both a pathological agent and an event – was going to require much more than medical expertise. This was partly because, far from pronouncing from a mountaintop, 'science' and 'medicine' rapidly and unwittingly reiterated themselves as messy, human activities, capable of generating as much uncertainty and ambiguity as concrete knowledge. In the UK, for example, an odd, self-appointed 'Independent SAGE' group established itself as a critical shadow of the government's official Scientific Advisory Group for Emergencies, amid claims that the latter was untransparent and politically compromised. But the need and desire for knowledge that was more-than-medical also came from a frank awareness that the things we needed to know about COVID-19 required a different expertise and skillset; it required, for example, knowledge of the relationship between crisis, confinement and the likelihood of gender-based violence; it meant knowledge of the reasons why trying to prevent infection by deploying shame might have very bad unintended consequences; it meant knowing what happens every day in a place like a museum, or a hospital, and how people working in these institutions can sometimes play an unsung role in the production and management of public feeling.

This work necessitated a temporal shift. For scholars doing the kind of work we gather together here – which is only a small slice of the critical humanities research that took place, in a similar spirit, in and around the pandemic – interpretation and meaning were no longer operationalised in reflective mode, or when the dust settled. Rather, they were instruments for making the crisis visible and resolvable, even as it was underway. This meant not only moving from a backwards-looking reflective stance to in-the-moment knowledge production, but also a shift in the time of research itself (Baraitser and Salisbury, 2020). Making an ongoing infectious disease crisis knowable meant setting aside longstanding commitments of many in the humanities community to *slow* research, to sometimes painstaking textual or archival methods, to checking, double-checking and triple-checking sources, to envisioning research impact over a span of many years – and a turn instead to approaches that were often immediate, scrappy, messy. And if we don't wish to revive, too much, a dusty cliché about slow-moving humanities professors poring over their equally dusty books (this, of course, has long been upended not least by scholars in environmental and medical humanities, in Black humanities, in computational humanities, among many other areas), we nonetheless argue that there is something distinctive about humanities researchers working in this crisis mode to make a health crisis knowable and visible, however imperfectly, with whatever tools they had to hand. This volume resists, therefore, a broader political project of devaluation aimed at the humanities; such a project, we argue, is inextricable from the governmental failures at knowledge-building – and harm reduction more broadly –that many of our chapters trace.

That last reference to tools is a reminder, finally, of another distinctive feature of these chapters, which is their relationship to methodological and technical innovation. In the chapters that follow, such innovation ranges from the use of animation to help bus passengers make sense of their exposure to the virus while getting around on public transport; to collaborating with user communities and engineers to create a wearable headset that would make a newly touchless environment perceptible to deafblind people; to using experimental film methods that foreground participation and the archiving of experience, in order to make a film that doesn't simply record experiences of racism, but becomes a site for political action and change. What is critical here is that none of these innovations, collaborations or novel methodological decisions are made for their own sake – it's not a facile logic of novelty that animates these projects. Rather, each chapter shows how the different authors filled the methodological gap between the expertise, knowledge and skills they had, on the one hand; and the need to make – with some rapidity – the unknowable known, on the other. This might mean drawing in new collaborators, risking a half-understood engagement with a technical object near to hand, or committing project resources (time, money, credibility) to some new technique with outputs that were, as yet, uncertain. There is here again a risk of drawing comparison with a now outmoded vision of humanities research, which in fact has been open to technological development and interdisciplinarity for some time (and indeed has been rendered open to this vision, whether it wishes it or not, by the remorseless financial and epistemic logic of the contemporary university). Nonetheless, we *do* want to claim that there is something distinctive in these chapters' willingness to take often rather large methodological risks – a willingness occasioned by the unfamiliar 'crisis' conditions within which the research was being conducted.

Chapter 1 is a critical reflection on a series of public health films created by a research team – Charlotte Veal, Paul Hurley, Emma Roe and Sandra Wilks, in collaboration with the filmmaker, Joseph Turp – on the subject of buses as spaces of more-than-human interactions and relationships, in the context of the COVID-19 virus. Structured as a conversation between Veal and Hurley, the piece focuses on the particular challenge of sensitising users to the unseen movement of microbes, without reproducing stigmatising imaginings of buses and bus travel as inherently or newly dangerous, dirty or contaminated. Equally, as the authors make clear, the project was committed to not representing (human) passengers in ways that either positioned them as threatening or isolated them artificially from non-human worlds. Many bus users, they argue, had already been acting in ways that acknowledge – if not always fully understand – their entanglement with buses as microbial environments, even on the briefest of journeys. In the work they undertook, the problem became one of how to effectively and faithfully communicate a complex set of considerations around communal hygiene and safety, at the same time as ensuring that the theoretical and methodological underpinnings of the research were uncompromised (and, indeed, developed) by the expedience of engaging audiences quickly and simply. By choosing to animate non-human elements of the bus (such as grab handles) with eyes and mouths, and overlaying short videos with conversations or monologues recorded by voice actors, the team repurposed a familiar genre for a theme more usually dominated by misleading or jarring characters and visual cues; for example, the 'microbe monster' favoured in advertisements for cleaning products. The seats, handles and windows which structure the environment of the bus became sites for discussion on how we are immersed in microbial worlds, and how the specific threat of COVID-19 within this immersion might be comprehended and forestalled.

In Chapter 2, Azadeh Emadi explores COVID-19 through the testimonies of deafblind people, a group for whom questions of knowledge and communication are frequently at the forefront of everyday navigation and experience. In the context of the pandemic, these questions became increasingly fraught. In the chapter, Emadi assembles a meticulous account of how their own research participants and those of their collaborators use touch to construct images and impressions of other people as well as their physical surroundings. This includes heightened attention to particular sources of information – such as the vibration of feet on a pavement – going far further than a logic of compensation, but instead opening up worlds of perception routinely disregarded by sighted people. With the problem of 'knowing' already seriously in contention, and with significant and systemic pre-existing barriers to relational health very much in place, COVID-19 and its responses structured deafblind people's experiences of public space in unsettling and disorienting ways. How did new rules around social distancing, for example, impact on interactions where touch had previously been key? How did altered uses of space – and an altered spatial relationship with other people – interrupt and distort the tangible and knowable world? Within these questions, Emadi outlines a challenge that moves across and beyond the peculiar circumstances of the pandemic: how to work with deafblind people to create a new technology of perception; in this case, a wearable headset or 'Touch Tool' which uses radar to process the immediate environment into information accessible to deafblind users. The aim of the Touch Tool is to offer an unobtrusive enhancement to the mosaic of impressions that the project's participants use to visualise objects and people in their surroundings. Research in the humanities, this chapter shows, can be crucial to the development of novel sensory innovations; in making the everyday experiences of deafblind people more problematic, the COVID-19 pandemic has helped provide the rationale for technology with the potential to be genuinely transformative.

Chapter 3 addresses a related but different set of questions around interactions with technology, asking how devices which rapidly became commonplace in the pandemic – in this instance, home (or workplace) lateral flow test (LFT) kits to indicate the presence of viral load – have been used, communicated and understood. Applying evidence from a panel of users and best-practice principles in communication design to the instructions that accompany LFTs, Sue Walker, Josefina Bravo and Al Edwards identify a crucial tension in what comprises 'good' instructions. Regulatory frameworks, the authors note, require compulsory information to be communicated alongside tests; the forms these communications take, however, are shaped by requirements (such as liability management) which are unnecessary for, and at times constraining of, the aim of relating easily comprehensible instructions quickly to almost anyone. 'Good' instructions, here, are a category very much open to contestation and nuance, and the authors assemble a powerful case for what testing instructions rooted in knowledge of how people actually process and respond to those instructions might look like. In some respects, this chapter crystallises one of the central contentions of the volume (and, indeed, the wider series). Amid repeated references to 'following the science' (and statements on the scale of their success), politicians lauded (and extensively funded) mass testing programmes. While enumerations of 'tests distributed' or 'tests traced' were key markers of political value, the unknown – and unknowable – figure of 'tests taken correctly' exerts a greater claim to salience. This figure is contingent, to a considerable degree, on how instructions were communicated and received; and understanding, critiquing and improving these processes is a matter requiring expertise from the arts and humanities. If, as the authors assert, there is likely to be a significant legacy of relatively simple tests taken by laypeople in non-clinical settings (processes already underway, for example, in the management of chronic illness), then the questions they identify here, on how such tests are demonstrated and explained – and how users, consequently, will engage with them – are of decisive importance.

At stake here are questions of communication, which are also a focus for Alison Blunt, Kathy Burrell, Georgina Endfield, Miri Lawrence, Eithne Nightingale, Alastair Owens, Jacqueline Waldock and Annabelle Wilkins, who take as their point of departure the UK Government's injunction to 'stay home', a public health strategy mirrored in a number of international contexts. What kind of home, Chapter 4 provokes us to ask, did these injunctions imagine? And how were homes inhabited or dwelled within, both easily and uneasily, not just as (largely) private households, but as wider emotional geographies which take in streets, neighbourhoods and public spaces? Making extensive use of testimonies taken from a diverse group of participants across the cities of Liverpool and London, the authors analyse how different people in different contexts connected with their surroundings in new ways, developing a firmer sense of place; how they negotiated feelings of loneliness that were rooted to the materiality and geography of home, transforming what might have previously been positive emotions around solitary living; how migration made room for attachments to multiple 'homes', with new barriers to mobility during COVID-19 imposing conflicting feelings of belonging and homesickness; how (even just visual) access to greenery and bodies of water made seclusion more bearable; and how racist attributions of the spread of disease pulled relatively secure feelings of home into crisis. In creating the conditions for home-workers, unemployed people and people on furlough to speak back to the injunction to 'stay home', the authors work towards a speculative and capacious idea of what home is and could be, in and for public health. In so doing, this chapter suggests that the diversity, complexity and inequity of experiences of home have to be taken seriously in future public health messages and interventions. Responses to new crises which rely on a homogenised and sanitised vision of home, and which ask us to 'stay home' without any deeper interrogation of what that might mean, will be insufficient to address both primary and secondary sources of harm.

Chapter 5 moves beyond our focus – broadly on technology and communication – up to this point, alighting on the specific context of the museum sector to untangle the role of emotions about and at work in the particular challenges faced by managers, curators, visitor guides and front-of-house staff. While this is in part an analysis of sectoral adaptation and adversity, Elizabeth Crooke and David Farrell-Banks, focusing empirically on Northern Ireland, move between macro- and microscopic lenses, using oral testimonies to explore complex emotional, political, economic and social situations and processes (such as furlough, precarity and shifting professional identities). COVID-19, the authors argue, exposed deep and long fissures in the museum sector; both individual and institutional priorities were crystallised by the pressures of shifting museums from physical to online spaces, collecting pandemic artefacts as a direct act of history-making and memorialisation, and continuing to offer formal and informal systems of care to audiences and staff. For Crooke and Farrell-Banks, the emotional attachment that museum staff had to their work – though not an unclouded phenomenon – acted primarily as a protective factor in navigating professional, personal and political changes and uncertainties. A renewed sense of purpose, too, could work against the nexus of painful emotions, such as loneliness, fear, anxiety and grief, which were wider products of the pandemic and the UK Government's preparedness and response. Amid attempts by the workers they interview to assemble a collective archive of the pandemic, Crooke and Farrell-Banks take the processes of collection and curation – and the welter of emotions, experiences and feelings that surround them – as the subject of their own project of preservation, ensuring that they are not simply allowed to fade from view.

Where earlier – and later – chapters in this volume address the novel context of COVID-19, Lesley Murray, Amanda Holt and Jessica Moriarty's Chapter 6 repositions our understanding of crisis in relation to the pandemic, posing it instead as a watershed moment in bringing previously ignored stories of suffering to the surface. The authors argue that the much-reported spike in gender-based violence (GBV) at the beginning of the pandemic allows for a more widespread – but still partial – questioning of whom GBV narratives exclude and make invisible. With GBV against women over the age of 50 frequently (mis)categorised as elder abuse (a conceptual framework that, the authors argue, misses important nuances in gender, power and mobility), this chapter identifies a narrative vacuum around older victims of GBV, with serious cultural, individual and legal consequences. While their broader research mobilises creative methodologies to encourage such stories to emerge, Murray, Holt and Moriarty's contribution to this volume focuses on two composite narratives of women in their eighties, assembled from multiple testimonies collected by the charity AGE UK. These stories draw together complex themes of abuse, control and constraint, first in a long narrative of physical and emotional violence over 57 years of marriage, and secondly in a shorter scenario of an abusive adult child returned to the family home. With COVID-19 present as the catalyst for these stories (but not their context), we can only speculate on how these dynamics might have contorted or sharpened, as – among a number of other determinants which make GBV more likely – physical proximity was increasingly enforced. Murray, Holt and Moriarty's chapter can also be read as a companion piece to Chapter 4 on the subject of home; indeed, it would be hard to draw out how the vision of home-as-sanctuary implicit in public health communications could be more strikingly subverted and compromised.

The problem of finding ways to preserve and communicate experiences which might otherwise have been rendered invisible is also a major focus of Anandi Ramamurthy and Ken Fero's Chapter 7 on 'obstinate memory'. Reflecting on the theories and methods behind their 2022 documentary, *Exposed*, on Black, Brown and migrant nurses and midwives' experiences of racism, the authors show how longer histories of racism in the National Health Service (NHS) were reformulated within the specific contingencies of COVID-19. Exposure, here, takes on several meanings: in the ways that racialisation contributed to how health workers were put in the way of viral and psychological harm; in the value of a 'documentary of force' approach in bringing such harms to light; and in the vulnerability of telling painful stories, and being cast in the difficult role of complainant. By attending closely to pasts and futures, Ramamurthy and Fero add new dimensions to what – at least for readers of other chapters in this volume – will be an increasingly familiar story. In their nuanced and perceptive piece, the COVID-19 pandemic stands not as something wholly new, but as a crisis which has landed in ways that follow deep and wide fault lines that were already well established in the UK in 2019. Anti-racist humanities work, their research attests, is sorely needed in the present: to untangle how structural racism (and the systemic devaluation of Black and Brown lives) plays out in specific institutional cultures and contexts, becoming encoded in responses to new emergencies and disasters. Their research also shows the power of creating an archive for, and a documentary to convey, testimonies which show precisely how this has occurred, in order to work backwards against racist exposure to multiple harms in future iterations of an NHS both in and out of crisis. Obstinate memory, this chapter suggests, is a technique not just of recognition, but of survival.

Chapter 8 in this volume, Fred Cooper, Luna Dolezal and Arthur Rose's essay on vaccine shaming, also takes sight at how particular lives and deaths have been invested with varying degrees of value (Fred Cooper is additionally an editor of the present volume, and an author of this introduction). Although there is a shared border here – vaccine uptake has usually been lower in racialised groups, in part because of a historical (and understandable) lack of trust in medical interventions and services – this chapter is concerned with acute (rather than chronic) dynamics of shame and marginalisation. What happens, the authors ask, when a shamed population is rapidly brought into being, specifically around non-conformity to public health initiatives; when members of that group are subsequently held accountable for a raft of negative outcomes (high infection and mortality rates, ongoing restrictions to everyday life and their own suffering and death); and when a crisis or disaster is publicly seen to be primarily affecting people who share culpability for their own illness? Bringing their research on shame and shaming into close proximity with Achille Mbembe's concept of necropolitics and Judith Butler's work on grievability, Cooper, Dolezal and Rose explore how shameful deaths are created and discussed, and the kinds of political decisions and omissions they make possible. COVID-19, they argue, significantly raised the stakes on vaccine 'hesitancy' and 'refusal', with public health communications on vaccination often heightening the burden of shame. In this context, internet users made new, 'anti-persuasive' forums, in the form of online spaces to shame and deride notable anti-vaxxers who had subsequently contracted COVID-19 and died, assembling in the process an accidental archive of the experience of dying of the disease. Beyond the immediate context of the COVID-19 pandemic, this chapter sensitises us to the complex workings of shame, and the damaging consequences of public health messaging which sets out to leverage this difficult emotion. Future pandemics will require mass vaccination programmes, and not everyone will co-operate. Likewise, other emergencies will be inflected with differing valuations of life. As normative judgements over 'good' and 'bad' behaviour are heightened, shame is likely to play a significant part.

The chapters that follow are in some ways a record of what it meant to do humanities research at a moment of crisis – to, in some cases, wholly re-orient an existing research agenda towards an as-yet-uncovered piece of the pandemic puzzle. There will be space in the years ahead for thinking more carefully – perhaps more critically – about the epistemic politics of this moment, and the inevitable instrumentalisation of research agendas that it entailed. In this volume, however, and in its companions, we want to make space for recording the rigorous epistemological force of the humanities during COVID-19. While the focus of this series of volumes has necessarily been on work (primarily) taking place in the humanities, for reasons detailed at length in the preface, it nonetheless takes sight at disciplinary practices with fluid and porous borders, and resonance far beyond the spaces they originated in; most notably, we suspect, for scholarship in public health and science and technology studies. This is a diverse and eclectic set of chapters pitched at a broad readership, intended to provide a frame of reference for research on COVID-19 – and emerging or ongoing crises and their epistemologies – well into the future. At a time of ongoing political and bureaucratic attack – as we write, some hundreds of humanities colleagues in the UK alone are under threat of redundancy, while early career colleagues are casually tossed aside – this volume also stands as a testament to what humanities research can do, what it *does* do, acknowledging the expertise, care and skill that scholars in philosophy, literature studies, history, media, human geography and so many other areas used to make the pandemic knowable.

References

Baraitser, L. and Salisbury, L. (2020), 'Containment, delay, mitigation': Waiting and care in the time of a pandemic [version 2; peer review: 2 approved]. *Wellcome Open Research*, 5(129). doi: 10.12688/wellcomeopenres.15970.2

Bunn, S. (2021), Mass testing for COVID-19: January update on lateral flow tests, Parliamentary Office of Science and Technology. Available at: https://post.parliament.uk/mass-testing-for-covid-19-january-update-on-lateral-flow-tests/ (accessed 8 May 2023).

Cartwright, L. (1995), *Screening the Body: Tracing Medicine's Visual Culture*. Minneapolis, MN: University of Minnesota Press.

Cooper, F., Dolezal, L. and Rose, A. (2023), *Covid-19 and Shame: Political Emotions and Public Health in the UK*. London: Bloomsbury.

Halpern, O. (2014), *Beautiful Data: A History of Vision and Reason since 1945*. Durham, NC: Duke University Press.

Latour, B. (1987), *Science in Action: How to Follow Scientists and Engineers through Society*. Cambridge, MA: Harvard University Press.

Rheinberger, H.-J. (1997), *Towards a History of Epistemic Things: Synthesizing Proteins in the Test Tube*. Stanford, CA: Stanford University Press.

1

Pandemic imaginaries of interspecies relatedness: More-than-human microbial methods on the bus

Charlotte Veal, Paul Hurley, Emma Roe and Sandra Wilks

The study of human–non-human relations, within a conceptual framework that decentres human exceptionalism (Menon and Karthik, 2017) and challenges the nature–society separation with its legacy of presenting the natural world as somehow 'out there', has gained traction within the social sciences and humanities (Büscher, 2022; Greco, 2022; Haraway, 2016; Whatmore, 2006; 2017). This body of work has started to reconceive ecological politics through mapping out how humans are situated in complex social relations with biological and physical worlds. Lively discussions have ensued, foregrounding multispecies geographies (Gillespie and Collard, 2015), vitalist ecologies (Bennett, 2010; Braun, 2015), and post-humanist theorising of more-than-human entanglements (Anderson, 2014; Wolfe, 2010). Within this field, the study of human–non-human relations has been dominated by well-established cultural interest areas; for example, animals, foodstuff and plants. There is also work that engages with non-human aspects of planetary life that is harder to grapple with due to the temporality, spatiality and inhuman materiality of multispecies worlds, such as the geological (Clark and Yusoff, 2017). Social studies of the microbial sit between these points of human–non-human scholarship. Viruses, bacteria, archaea, fungi and protists are methodologically trickier to study within social relations as they are challenging to witness as material, recognisable everyday objects in relation to human practices. And yet the COVID-19 pandemic demonstrated how the very real threat of infection was accompanied by multifarious imaginings of microbial agency and risk that radically changed everyday life.

Over the last two decades, social and economic anxieties associated with antimicrobial resistance, food and zoonotic disease risk, as well as the recent pandemic, have prompted a surge in social and cultural studies of the microbial (Hinchliffe and Bingham, 2008; Hinchliffe et al., 2018; Mather and Marshall, 2011) and the human microbiome (Greenhough et al., 2020). This literature brings attention to the vitality, materiality and dynamism of microbial life, when operating in assemblage with other non-humans – air, water, architecture, etc., co-producing worlds beyond human control (see Bosco, 2006; Hinchliffe and Whatmore, 2017; Whatmore, 2017). Human existence is always a more-than-human achievement (Greenhough, 2014; see also Latour, 1993; Stengers, 1997). Unlike the conceptual and theoretical developments, methodological developments to cater for the challenges of studying specific human–non-human relations have not kept pace. There is urgent need for further development of more-than-human methods that support sensing, understanding and 'doings' *with* microbial worlds, to add to existing work in this field (Dowling et al., 2017; see also Adams et al., 2021; Buller, 2015; Hodgetts and Lorimer, 2015; Swanson, 2017). This chapter addresses this absence, outlining the critical imperative for methodological innovation capable of advancing novel representations and literacies around interspecies relatedness.

Amidst calls to develop new techniques that 'allow us to engage with diverse and multiple worlds and non-human agencies' (Greenhough, 2014: 101), this chapter advances a more-than-human microbial methodology, using the example of public health videos created during the recent pandemic. Taking the lead from geography's 'creative turn' in research methods (Veal and Hawkins, 2020), the more-than-human microbial methodology presented here draws on three bodies of literature: filmmaking as research; affect theory; and artistic microbial methods. Participatory videos and filmmaking can work against and beyond text (Garrett, 2011; Jacobs, 2013) and are argued to better attune to the more-than-human dimensions of life (Lorimer, 2010; Richardson-Ngwenya, 2014). Others have put forward affect and emotion as informing cognition, behaviours and socio-political interactions in ways that may not be fully perceptible (Anderson, 2006; Gregg and Seigworth,

2010). Affect is central to the production of 'non-human charisma' (Lorimer, 2017) while emotions shape human relations to worlds unseen but sensed (Roe et al., 2021). Scholarly interest in the unfolding of social worlds through emotions, affects, practices and multisensual forces has found synergies with artistic approaches to microbial research that illustrate other ways of knowing and communicating the micro-scale (see Evans and Lorimer, 2021; Macduff et al., 2017). An important contribution from Roe et al. (2019) foregrounds aesthetics and imaginaries in illustrating microbial interactions *with* humans in the act of infection. Such work advocates for non-anthropogenic modes of researching *with* microbial worlds and attending to the material and imaginative, subtle and dynamic, forces they engineer (see Hinchliffe et al., 2005). The COVID-19 pandemic signals a critical imperative to develop microbial literacy (see Timmis et al., 2019). By microbial literacy the authors refer to the social and cultural knowledges and values that shape non-specialist publics' *encounters* with medico-scientific information about microbial communities and their risk. And it involves attuning to how individuals and different community groups (whether by age, race, ethnicity, class, etc.) *apply* information about microbial risk (hazard identification, sources of infection, strategies of prevention, care of self or other, etc.) to their routines and practices in ordinary settings and everyday life.

The main portion of this chapter is framed around a conversation that took place on the video calling platform Zoom between co-investigator and artist-academic Paul Hurley (PH) and co-investigator and landscape scholar Charlotte Veal (CV) in April 2022 as part of the project Routes of Infection, Routes to Safety: Understanding Risk and the Viral Imagination on Public Transport; they are two members of a four-person research team. The other two members were principal investigator and cultural geographer Emma Roe and co-investigator and microbiologist Sandra Wilks. The thoughts and ideas expressed in Veal and Hurley's conversation reflect and relay hours of discussion between the whole team during the project. Roe and Wilks have co-authored ideas central to this chapter, discussed and edited it. Work on developing this chapter was part of the post-research reflection, evaluation and project write-up phase that included a stakeholder report (Roe et al., 2021), participatory workshops with research participants and an Arts and Humanities Research Council (AHRC) evaluative summary. A reflexive conversation, central to the collaborative model of working throughout the project, seemed an appropriate written form to share the team's methodological experimentations. Deliberately dialogical, the chapter raises questions about how stories of the trials and tribulations of research, particularly in fast-paced and fluctuating socio-political and scientific contexts, are told. Lightly edited, the format is also intended to be provocative and free flowing, creating a *reflective* exploratory space to think about and push thinking on the more-than-human and microbial methods specifically.

Routes to Safety's aim was to understand the personal application of infection prevention measures beyond clinical settings and to build confidence in bus travel during a time when public transport use was being discouraged (for example, by Transport Secretary Grant Shapps, quoted in Davies, 2020). The field work included ethnography and semi-structured research interviews (between January and October 2021). The team, on the request of UK Research and Innovation (UKRI), made a commitment that more than 50 per cent of research participants would be drawn from members of Black, Asian or Minority Ethnic (BAME) communities in order to capture the disproportionate impact the pandemic was having on BAME communities (Public Health England, 2020a). Hence, from the outset the team established a collaboration with the Bristol Somali Youth forum who helped recruit from their community. The project concluded with producing four animated films with public health messaging, grouped under the title 'You're Never Alone on the Bus', with filmmaker Joseph Turp.

The chapter reflects on the processes of concept-inception, team-discussion and dissemination-reception of these films to/by various audiences. It argues that developing novel representations and literacies around interspecies relatedness in shared public spaces like the bus is vital to facilitating new understandings not only of human–microbial relations in the context of COVID-19, but also how more-than-human methods might be applicable to infection prevention campaigns during future public health challenges (winter colds, flu, norovirus) and knowledge-making around other global health challenges such as antimicrobial resistance. It is structured under four sub-headings: context for the film; microbial aesthetics;

politics of microbial aesthetics; and scriptwriting, before concluding with a call for critically creative more-than-human microbial methods.

Context for the film

Charlotte Veal (CV): Paul, let's start with the background context for the public engagement dimension of the research project. This was a dual challenge underscored by UK Government COVID-19 messaging that, from the outset, warned the public against public transport use. On the one hand, many bus users expressed limited microbial literacy. On the other hand, because of a long history of stigmatising the bus as 'dirty' or a space utilised only by lower-income sectors of society (see TfL, 2012), our attempts to address this tension were met by bus operators' reluctance. Operators were hesitant to represent the microbial in their communications about infection prevention measures such as physical distancing, hand hygiene and mask wearing. Can you reflect on how the concept for the film developed within this context and who was involved?

Paul Hurley (PH): So, we had a filmmaker on board from the outset, Joseph Turp. Joe had worked with the research team on Mapping Microbes in 2016; a project that developed creative visualisations of surface transmission and hand hygiene in a mock-hospital ward (Roe et al., 2019). Joe was involved in the developmental phase of Routes to Safety and this helped coordinate our thinking on outputs. The team met regularly with Joe to discuss initial findings and how we might translate them into visual and informational materials around infection prevention. Discussions focused on ethnographic findings onboard buses and at bus stops – observing passenger behaviours, social interactions and mundane encounters with bus architecture – as well as initial interviews with bus drivers and bus users (beginning in April 2021).

CV: The creative process was also informed by our own pandemic-shaped everyday encounters with infection prevention and protection: by things that we'd heard from friends; by our experiences of relatives being hospitalised and of children being in school; by those daily interactions that felt 'new'; and by the negotiations that we were having with the 'virus' through ordinary tasks like catching a bus, going to the supermarket or inviting someone into our home.

PH: The ideas for the films came out of our own lived reality that we were simultaneously researching. It was a very dynamic situation and while the team planned to do something like the Mapping Microbes project, it became clear that Routes to Safety needed to look beyond surface transmission to consider airborne transmission. The aesthetic of our UV-lit microbial worlds created during Mapping Microbes also bore an uncanny resemblance to some public information films released by Public Health England (2020b). We pledged to continue innovating rather than to rehearse the same approach.

CV: The creative process also had to engage constructively with people's everyday lived experiences of a rapidly evolving medical and political context and the associated affective and emotional forces cultivated under the framework of government public health messaging which enhanced a sense of risk.

PH: When research began in January 2021, the team had to go through an intensive process of ethical and health and safety approval to travel on buses. It's strange to think now about the intensity of anxiety and perceived risk from boarding a bus. Back then, we were in a very different reality. It was a challenging context to be working in. And yet that challenge also created a richness of disturbance to our conceptual and methodological working from which to creatively respond. The ordinary had been shaken up to such a degree by this unknown microbial non-human that we needed a new method of research. One question the team kept returning to was how to map out the new practices that were ever emerging in this new reality. Unlike the more familiar pathogens we had been thinking with in Mapping Microbes, the scientific understanding of SARS-CoV-2 was ever-evolving.

CV: Did this 'unnerving' and 'new' pandemic context mean that you developed a more experimental relationship to your creative practice as a performance artist and community research facilitator?

PH: There was certainly an unknownness that I and the team were encountering as the once familiar bus environment was rendered strange. Also, hospital infection prevention practices and behaviours we'd previously studied were starting to become more ordinary as people performed and experienced them on the bus.

It felt like there was an opportunity to do something different, but we couldn't be as artistically experimental as we might have been, in a less pressured window of time. Tens of thousands of people were dying and this intervention we were trying to make was attempting to seriously address the practices that gave people more susceptibility to contracting the virus, while also helping the country safely get back to more normal levels of social and economic activity.

CV: The starting point for the films was the challenge of representing the SARS-CoV-2 virus in ways that were scientifically sound but equally engaging and accessible. Elsewhere, Bioart has given form to microbes as part of enquiries into biological worlds (Kelley, 2016; Mitchell, 2015) and visualisations have supported pedagogic training among healthcare workers (Macduff et al., 2017). What seemed missing were social *behaviours* in response to microbes.

Looking at the films made (the reader can find them here: www.neveraloneonthebus.org/outputs/), what is striking is the absence of human characters. Instead, the bus architecture does the talking. Where did the idea of bus-architecture characters come from and what was their role in the films?

PH: Experimenting in more-than-human microbial methods was exciting, but also difficult. Part of that difficulty was ethical. When scriptwriting began in spring 2021, restrictions were being eased, the winter lockdown had ended, and face coverings were still advised in many indoor contexts. Older people and those with certain clinical vulnerabilities had been offered the vaccine. But there was beginning to be, as I remember it, more slippage in how guidance and regulations were being communicated and followed. Bus passengers recounted tensions around some people wearing or not wearing masks, some passengers wanting to open the windows while others wanted to close them because it was cold. A key parameter for the team was to not reinforce prejudices around who was performing certain behaviours judged as riskier or behaviours that intensified risks for others. We didn't want to be didactic or judgemental about these practices.

And so, the team asked, 'What *can* we do?' if we don't want to have human characters in the films, if it's not about something like one-upmanship: 'Oh, I'm wearing a mask'. That's quite a simplistic, potentially problematic and stigmatising scenario to adopt, and attitudes towards mask-wearing were (and remain) fluid. Joe did some initial sketches around the bus itself being a character and Joe and I did some photographic and video experiments at the bus depot, with the bus doors being like the mouth and trying to think of the horizontal opening windows as eyelids. We explored thinking about the architecture of the bus as a character that helped us visualise different kinds of agents, including – drawing upon Haraway (2008) and Whatmore (2006) – non-human agents. The scenario of infection is often framed as being between humans (unwashed hands, coughs and sneezes, poor food preparation), but in this project the research team approached the 'event' of infection as being an encounter between humans, surfaces, air, the virus and other microbes. Each has agency and is actively entangled in the event of transmission or infection (drawing on geographers writing on relations and entanglements; Allen, 2012; Lorimer, 2010; Taylor and Pacini-Ketchabaw, 2018).

CV: Anthropomorphic characters such as cartoonish representations of 'germ monsters' are not uncommon in the visual language of public health. What did feel visually new was how the bus characters focused discussions towards *practices* onboard the bus like cleaning or ventilation that affect the atmosphere and environment of the bus. Making characters out of the bus architecture visually detracted responsibility away from the individual human and foregrounded relationality in an ever-evolving bus environment with other humans, non-humans and microbes. This was closer to the socio-technoscientific reality of entangled human relations with complex and diverse microbial communities, rather than a narrative of fixed and oppositional relations represented by the UK Government's (and various strategies taken by devolved nations) attempts to 'control the virus' or to fight a 'war against COVID' (Waylen, 2021: n.p.).

PH: Each of the films – *Fresh Air Shows You Care*, *Use Your Head to Stop the Spread*, *Leave Some Space Just in Case*, and *Keep Your Micro-Passengers to Yourself* – focused on a scenario that had been reported in our interviews, such as sitting next to someone who was coughing or somebody closing the bus window rather than opening it for ventilation. And that's when the bus characters came in – like Sammy STOP Button and Backseat

Bob – with supporting human characters who were largely off screen. Joe started writing the scripts and the research team went back and forth, redrafting and editing, via collaborative online documents. Through the bus characters, stories of human–non-human interactions were told.

CV: This is particularly evident in one of the films where a trio of grab handles became commentators for the off-screen action of a human walking down the stairs and sneezing (Figure 1.1).

PH: The viewer doesn't see the sneezing human character, but does see the interaction between these non-human characters; this gave a useful distance from the 'responsibilisation of individuals' in transmission of the virus and yet somehow also points to the collective responsibility of bus passengers. Aesthetically it links to a long history in animation – Disney's 1940 *Fantasia*, ITV's 1984 *Thomas the Tank Engine*, Pixar's 2008 *WALL-E* – of objects becoming animated characters, and with the animation style that uses a mixture of hand-drawn and stop motion mixed with live action. The more-than-human methodological approach innovated was driven by a desire to find a format that allowed us to not characterise, or stereotype, the identity of who may be inclined to follow, or not follow, infection prevention advice.

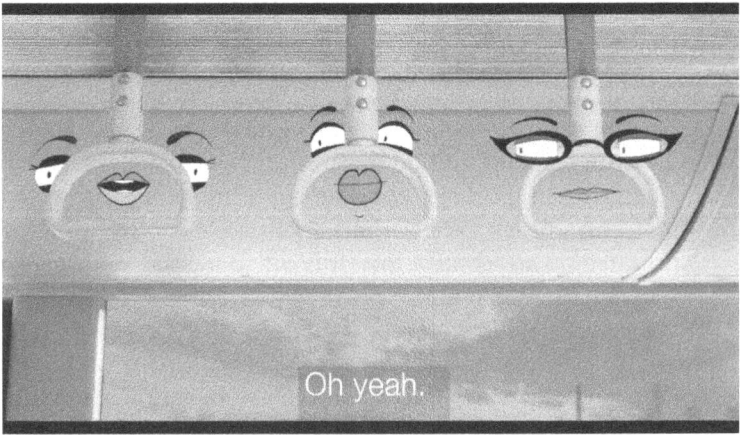

Figure 1.1 Still from *Use Your Head to Stop the Spread* (short video), part of the 'You're Never Alone on the Bus' series (© 2021 Joseph Turp and Routes to Safety. All rights reserved.)

Microbial aesthetics

CV: Thinking back to the visual cultures of the pandemic (see Lynteris, 2020: 190) and UK Government public health films especially, the decision *not* to focus on humans was, aesthetically speaking, substantially different. Co-producing four shorter films, however, echoed the stylistics that the various UK regional governments were working with.

PH: To make four shorter films was a practical choice, to do with distribution. If these films were to be shown (as they were) on social media, or on buses, then they needed to be short, because people's viewing concentration is much reduced on those platforms. And while these four films were 'of a piece', part of a series, they also each stood alone. Each has a different story that reinforces a collective message. For example, they certainly started off being very short words, punchy tag lines like 'Hands – Face – Space'.

CV: And there was a simple visual design – icons, simple text – and a limited colour palette like blue and white, connecting to NHS visual design.

PH: By 2021, the various UK goverments started to do longer pieces; some about air and meeting people indoors including one showing a cloud of particles spreading in a room where people were sitting.[1] I remember pandemic imagery featured representations of sticky yucky stuff (potential virus on surfaces), of neon clouds or ectoplasm (potential airborne virus) being spread about in a domestic environment. Such images were loaded with affect (unsettling, fear, disgust, etc.) that leveraged emotional reactions conducive to coercing individuals into adopting 'responsible' behaviours through the 'yuk' factor (see Allen, 2021). These were the dominant representations of the virus circulating in the world.

CV: Finding new tools and techniques to communicate non-human worlds that affirm their agency without provoking fear and disgust seems like an important step for addressing the lacuna of microbial literacy among non-specialist publics.

PH: In the films in the series, 'Never Alone on the Bus', there's something more light-hearted and immediately kind of playful. A couple of participants said that there's something child-like about the films; like a *Thomas the Tank Engine* world where bits of the bus talk to each other. Perhaps animating the non-human in that way, making that imaginative leap to give the non-human a character, creates a frivolousness or playfulness to it, that was understandably absent from government communications. We would see humans talking, a minister sharing stark messages, and very naturalistic home environments with humans acting in a naturalistic manner with a spooky invisible layer of infection present. Because our team doesn't work for a public health body, we had licence to try to engage people in a different way.

CV: This microbial imaginary equally rejects images of microscopy or anthropomorphic representations of microbial 'monsters' that have historically been mobilised. These, of course, can be helpful, but also affectively alienating and can misinform people about microbial behaviour and how this connects to practices of infection prevention. Can you say something more about the microbial non-human and the practicalities of working on this with Joe?

PH: Alongside animating bus architecture, a key parameter for the films was to visualise the microbial community of the bus, which is both viral and bacterial. The research team's microbiome study (as yet unpublished) evidenced that the types of microbes on the bus are mostly environmental and are not a risk to human health. Nevertheless, these are the microbial things that we are often scared of interacting with because we can't see them. This invisibility felt important. A challenge of the project was that the world, for many, changed radically because of new knowledge of the presence of a non-human agent – SARS-CoV-2. Unless we're microbiologists with a specialised electron microscope and access to the virus we can't see it. Most of us don't really understand what 'it' is or its viral character. This is a real societal challenge. How do we communicate something that people can't understand or get to know using their conventional sensory and talk-based approaches? Yet onboard the bus, people were doing all sorts of things to adapt their practices to the 'unknowable' virus.

CV: The once familiar space was rendered uncanny or distorted – by face masks, signage about where to sit, practices of physical distancing. People's everyday experience of the bus travelling space was altered by an unseen, but sensed, microbial world. For many bus users interviewed, this produced intense feelings of uncertainty that shaped interactions with other passengers, the bus architecture and the possibly present virus.

PH: The team wanted to work with findings from interviews, where passengers, drivers and cleaners were asked how they imagined the virus and how they thought they might catch it. People talked about what they thought the virus wanted, like 'it wants to survive', or 'it wants to infect people'. People were giving the virus agency. Incorporating this in the films in a way that wasn't alarmist was imperative, because one of the research aims was to inspire confidence on the bus. If people are carrying out infection prevention practices, the bus *is* a safe place. If they're not, then that becomes harder to say. We didn't want to reinforce government messaging that was targeting public transport as more risky than other indoor environments.

I remember Sandra Wilks, the microbiologist on the research team, has talked about adverts for domestic cleaning products where you have little 'germ monsters' trying to jump out of toilets, or by contrast adverts for food products that contain 'healthy bacteria' for the gut, visualised by a warm glow. Representing the virus as an individual, whether monster or protector, sat uncomfortably with the more-than-human methodology the research team was developing.

CV: In three of the films, the microbial is hinted at (coughs, sneeze), but it's the fourth – *Keep Your Micro-Passengers to Yourself* – where microbial representations begin to be untethered from this unhelpful good-bug bad-bug dichotomy. Could you explain how you worked aesthetically with the microbial in this film?

PH: A recurring theme of discussion was how to represent *communities* of microbes as biofilms on surfaces or as a combination of different bacteria and viruses and whatever else in the air. This was approached through a visual animation that was layered onto the film afterwards. It was a glittery glow that was around various bus surfaces. And these were also characters.

Lines were introduced into the script about what we called 'micro-pets' or 'micro-passengers' – to point to the invisible microbial communities that live in or on us. The non-human bus characters, like Sammy STOP Button, drawn by our character designer Adriana Meirelles, were aware of the microbial communities living on them. Some characters were happy about those communities and others were less so, which was reflective of human feelings about microbes. This is despite only a small proportion of the microbes in and around us being pathogenic, as our (unpublished) microbiome study results showed. But it was very difficult to bring these perspectives into the film. The fourth film is the one that tries to do that, and that was certainly the one that proved most difficult to write. It was also the film that met a certain amount of resistance from bus industry stakeholders. Bus passengers seemed warmer to it. They got it. But I think bus operators were concerned that this film portrayed buses in a bad light, reinforcing the stigma attached to them as 'dirty' and full of bacteria, which is a story they wanted to avoid. More-than-human methods can provoke thinking on microbial agency, but there are clearly ethical and political considerations when working with various stakeholders.

Politics of microbial aesthetics

CV: Could you say more about the wider politics of microbial aesthetics?

PH: The films were shot as a series of fixed camera shots of the bus interior, which was brightly lit. The bus company that hosted the filming was keen that we used the new buses. These were very smart and colourful. It's quite clean and bright. Different parts of the architecture, like the seats, STOP button and grab handles, were filmed and then had hand-drawn animation layered on in post-production; for instance, drawn eyes or a mouth which were animated over the live action video. The live action video bits were made up of actors drawn from the research team and research participants who had volunteered to sit in the background to give a sense of movement around the animated characters.

CV: The videos were quite cheery in their aesthetic. Exchanges between the bus architecture characters were conversational and chatty.

PH: This evoked the conviviality that many bus passengers valued but noted was lost during the pandemic. A range of voices was selected for the STOP button, the seat, etc.: different genders and ages, different ethnicities, different regional accents, again reflecting a diverse bus passenger and driver community.

CV: This diversity, from memory, was a response to wider literature that celebrated the bus as a multicultural space – of exchanges between unacquainted others (see Jensen, 2009; Wilson, 2011) – challenging the narrative of violence and racism on board or the social-spatial inequalities associated with these networks. And yet, interviewees affirmed the social and economic factors that were placing some bodies at greater risk of exposure to COVID-19; buses were a vital resource, transporting key workers to work, and our BAME interviewees to shops and health appointments.

PH: The routes we selected in which to conduct our ethnography also crosscut diverse neighbourhoods to acknowledge these social geographies.

When it came to the animated micro-passengers – an almost glittery sparkly twinkle – we wanted them to have a positive bright affectation, rather than a slimy feeling. It was something lively. It's about giving a sense that there are these communities and these worlds, that we can't see, that exist everywhere, including on the bus, but that's okay.

CV: Were there any concerns around anthropomorphising characters?

PH: The decision was made early on to make parts of the bus architecture characters rather than the microbes. Sammy STOP Button and Backseat Bob were intentionally anthropomorphised. We gave the bus architecture names and characters, knowing that people generally don't think of those things as having characters. Whereas people do think of a virus having a character – a character that was often framed in government messaging as a military adversary. Not anthropomorphising the virus troubles an individualisation of the virus as a monster, a singular 'thing'. That doesn't make sense in microbiological terms nor in how we might think of these communities of microbes and the way they interact with our own microbiome. Using the bus architecture as characters helped to give the film these stories. I am not sure if we did cute-ify them, but they remind me of *Creature Comforts*, an early Aardman Animations film (1989). Using those bits of architecture to tell the story of the human interaction with the microbial felt like a useful device to engage viewers in a story rather than just in an informational message.

CV: There was also something about how the bus characters became observers capable of reflecting on both worlds; the spectator and performer.

PH: In Greek tragedy, you'd have the chorus, or in Shakespearean theatre the narrator, who has greater knowledge of the drama on stage than the characters do. The narrator knows more about what's just happened or what's about to happen. They have this privileged position. I wonder if there's something in how the bus architecture is given a privileged position of knowledge because it can see what humans can't see, and in some of the films, the micro-pets.

Scriptwriting

CV: Creating public health resources that support confidence in public transport usage was a key aim of the project. What audiences did you trial the films with?

PH: Much of the social science field work involved interviewing bus drivers, bus cleaners and bus users. We chose to interview bus users solely from Bristol's Somali community, prompted by a condition of funding that at least 50 per centof participants originate from BAME groups, and by learning about the disproportionate impact of the pandemic on that community (Sayaqle, 2020). Some interviewees spoke of the challenge of UK Government pandemic communication materials being unavailable in different languages. Producing something that was accessible and that could be subtitled in different languages informed the creative process. The aesthetic was also oriented towards that – to try to be engaging and playful, rather than being reliant on linguistic understanding as the primary communicator. The team hoped the characters would be entertaining and relatable to different audiences. I'm not sure how effective that was because we haven't yet had them translated and subtitled in different languages.

Each of the films ended with a short slogan that relates to what's happened in the film. One film is about two bus seats talking about where passengers sit. At the end of the dialogue, they say, 'give some space, just in case'. This then comes up as a title. Again, when we screened the films with multilingual audiences of different ages, the feedback was that the narratives were engaging and the slogans were memorable.

CV: It feels timely to be exploring how more-than-human methods might support microbial literacy, but doing so in ways that are sensitive to the differentiated social and cultural understandings of the microbial, cleanliness, dirt and 'other'. Continuing the theme of cultural reference points, could you say more about the use of analogies and of creating personalities behind each character?

PH: In the film, *Use Your Head to Stop the Spread*, three dangling grab handles are talking about humans walking down the stairs, whether one of them is wearing a mask or not. The research team with Joe tried different versions of that script and kept coming up against this thing that we didn't want to do, of being judgemental about mask wearing. It was around the time of the European Football Cup and the project lead, Emma Roe, suggested running with football as a frame for the film. The dialogue between the handles became a sports commentary on human behaviour – of whether the person was going to catch their sneeze; they spot someone with a mask and that's one point. It has this sense of a sporting analogy, but also reminds me of games you play with children, of spotting things outside the window, of counting red cars to keep a child quiet on a long journey.

CV: Developing appropriate and relatable characters was arguably more important when it came to breath and breathing as with the film *Fresh Air Shows You Care*.

PH: Scientific research was increasingly emphasising the importance of fresh air, which got us thinking; okay, how do we communicate about breath and keeping windows open? Central to our thinking about indoor spaces was needing to breathe and so this character became a calming yoga-teacher-type voice that was talking about breathing clean air in. It was a shift away from a didactic or alarmist tone: 'You must keep the windows open'. Our yoga teacher, with a lovely calming positive voice, was able to say that it's good to breathe and it's good to have fresh air.

CV: None of the team are scriptwriters, including Joe – who's in the field of cinematography – and my academic and artistic background is in dance. How did the process of writing work?

PH: The research team used a shared online document for the scripts and sometimes we worked offline and sometimes we collectively edited it 'live'. It was a useful lesson to try to boil down these complex ideas, during a dynamic time when guidance was ever-shifting and when rules differed geographically according to political borders, into something that was a real kernel, in an exchange that wasn't heavy-handed. It wasn't about being didactic, but it did have a sort of educational function.

Collaborating on the script felt like a useful process in pushing the team's conceptual and methodological thinking. How do we do more-than-human research and communicate interspecies relatedness through film? How can that process of scriptwriting enrich and enliven practices of engaging other publics whether through policy reports (Roe et al., 2021) or through stakeholder workshops? There was something valuable in being able to consolidate these ideas into exchanges of short, simple sentences and dialogues. Other than the statements at the end of each film, which were in the 'official' authorial voice of the researchers, the rest of the dialogue came through exchanges between the characters.

CV: There were multiple non-human voices that were manifesting or conjuring some of the issues that we were looking at. It's interesting how removing a word or a sentence transformed the flow and meaning of a particular socio-microbiological issue, practice or relationship.

PH: The team were thinking about spoken text, in different voices, and so intonation and how we structure those sentences were also something we had to learn about. The scripts were sent to voice-over artists under Joe's direction, and we found they interpreted the meaning of the words slightly differently. Some words were changed because of the voiceover artist's natural way of speaking. Everyone has a different rhythm or cadence. Our words didn't quite fit in their mouths. During writing sessions, the team read them out loud, which felt quite strange, but it was necessary to get to know that material in a very intimate way. And it drew us out of formal modes of writing for academic or report-reading audiences, and towards experimenting with more accessible and engaging materials for communicating interspecies relations.

CV: Scriptwriting opened up avenues for the research team to apply dramatic writing techniques (scene heading, structure, pause, rhythm, intonation, dialogues) to co-produce knowledge (with non-human bus characters and micro-pets) about public health and disseminate information in visually appealing and affectively generative ways. Such devices have critical and creative force to engage audiences on a different level (to public health and scientific pedagogy) that is playful and imaginative, and which affirms the contingencies at play in the act of preventing infection.

Conclusion: for more-than-human microbial methods?

CV: The pandemic has been a profound testament to the multispecies worlds that we live in, and what exceeds human control and representation. Acknowledging the vitality, materiality and dynamism of more-than-human worlds – of microbes demonstrating agency that shapes human behaviour and practices – demands that scholars do research differently. To follow Dowling et al. (2017: 823), there is a lacuna of knowledge in how 'to engage, to embody, to image and imagine, to witness, to sense, to analyse – across, through, with, and as, more-than-humans'. Looking forward, where do you see the conceptual and creative methodological developments in contributing to this gap in doing interspecies research and communication?

PH: The first is around interdisciplinarity and the specific constellation of knowledges and practices that came together for this project. There is growing work examining more-than-human methods, but there is still less methodological innovation on social and cultural approaches to studying the microbial, with some exceptions (Lorimer et al., 2019). There is a pressing need to develop both methods and ways of thinking that combine socio-scientific with microbiological worlds to make knowable microbial communities and their behaviours – what's happening on surfaces and how their presence (or imagined presence) shapes interactions between human practices. Routes to Safety is a small step towards addressing this knowledge gap.

CV: Interdisciplinarity is, of course, not new in research. Routes to Safety amalgamated knowledges and practices from microbiology, geography, landscape architecture and performance art, and methods spanning scientific, social and creative techniques – including swabbing, interviews, ethnography and filmmaking. None of these methods were innovative in and of themselves but what was valuable in the context of the pandemic was the mutually informative process. Passenger concerns about where the virus might be located informed where swabbing took place, and decisions to swab particular surfaces informed the team's onboard observations as passengers touched or avoided surfaces.

PH: The more-than-human microbial methodology offers ways of thinking about bridging the gap between microbiological processes and social anxieties and practices around the imagined world shaping the actions of microbes. And I'm folding the filmmaking process in here too. While Joe didn't participate in the other research activities, he was involved in the interdisciplinary thinking-through-reflecting-and-talking sessions that were mutually informative and productive. These creative conversations helped iterate the content of the films and fed into the team's interdisciplinary grappling around many of the broader research aims and objectives.

CV: Part of that interdisciplinary more-than-human microbial contribution seems to be around activating other, more-than-representational, frames of knowing.

PH: This brings me to my second point. I think what the team has done is quite ambitious but also vital in terms of engaging – or helping to understand *how* to engage – people with the socio-ecological dimensions of contemporary life or the challenges of the contemporary moment. And especially people from multicultural backgrounds where linguistic considerations need to be enveloped into the methodological process and dissemination practices. Creative filmmaking and scriptwriting solicited playful aesthetics, the affective, the emotional, the imaginary –qualities that interviewees identified as driving infection prevention decision-making. The impetus for these forces weren't always rational or grounded in microbiological 'evidence', but did matter to the rationale and reasoning that drove decisions about when and how to travel, what practices and behaviours to adopt and how to negotiate risk and anxiety in the context of indoor spaces like the bus.

CV: More analysis is needed to determine how 'successful' the films were in building microbial literacy, but what they possibly offered was a different way of knowing and encountering the non-human – one that wasn't alarmist but conversational, playful.

PH: Storytelling (and other animation tools) by our non-human characters, with diverse accents and voices, disrupted traditionally dominant voices in public health films. And they also narrated more-than-human relationships involved in the process of infecting, which from my perspective asks us to think further about how we live alongside others. My creative approach was driven by a need to think differently about how bodies are interacting within the bus, as well as the interactions of human and non-human bodies (like viruses). The films offer ways for imagining and facilitating a space in which new knowledges can be made. Creative methods are one of the tools to be drawn on to respond to this pandemic and inevitable future health challenges because they enable a different perspective on our relationship to the world, especially human–non-human worlds.

Coda

Human–microbial relations have come under international attention, not only in political and policy settings but also in everyday spaces and within ordinary lives, in response to a range of microbial crises. There is a pressing need to develop concepts that afford greater sociomicrobial knowledges, and novel methods for studying the more-than-human, in ways that account for worlds where humans are not the sole force of change. In response, this chapter has applied posthumanist thinking and interspecies discourse to tell novel stories of infection prevention for multispecies living. It thought through the innovation of a creative more-than-human microbial method, in the form of four animated films, capable of supporting sense-making of the microbial and building microbial literacy in the context of infection prevention and protection in shared indoor spaces. In contrast to medico-scientific representations, the films worked against and beyond other textual forms of knowledge, communicating through forces that included aesthetics, affect, emotion, the imaginative and more-than-human storytelling that was playful and humorous. There is great potential for methodologies like this, not only in the field of infection prevention and communication, but in associated public health work in pandemics like COVID-19, in 'wicked problems' like antimicrobial resistance, and in socio-ecological crises both current and unknown.

Acknowledgements

The chapter is based on research that was funded by a UKRI AHRC COVID-19 Rapid Response Grant: AH/V014986/1 that ran from February 2021 to February 2022. We would like to thank Joseph

Turp and Adriana Meirelles for their creative contributions. A special thanks to Mohamed Abdi Sayaqle and Somali Youth Voice for their steadfast support and the time they gave to the research. We also wish to thank our industry partners First Bus, Bluestar and Dawn Badminton-Capps of Bus Users UK.

Note

1 See www.youtube.com/watch?v=qYZMOG2kUWg

References

Adams, M., Ormrod, J. and Smith, S. (2021), Notes from a field: A qualitative exploration of human–animal relations in a volunteer shepherding project. *Qualitative Research*, 23(1).

Allen, B. (2021), Emotion and COVID-19: Toward an equitable pandemic response. *Journal of Bioethical Inquiry*, 18(3), 403–406.

Allen, J. (2012), A more than relational geography? *Dialogues in Human Geography*, 2(2), 190–193.

Anderson, B. (2006), Becoming and being hopeful: Towards a theory of affect. *Environment and Planning D: Society and Space*, 24(5), 733–752.

Anderson, K. (2014), Mind over matter? On decentring the human in Human Geography. *Cultural Geographies*, 21(1), 3–18.

Bennett, J. (2010), *Vibrant Matter: A Political Ecology of Things*. Durham, NC: Duke University Press.

Bosco, F. J. (2006), 'Actor-Network Theory, Networks, and Relational Approaches in Human Geography' in S. Aitken and G. Valentine (eds), *Approaches to Human Geography*. Sage: London, pp.136–146.

Braun, B. (2015), 'From Critique to Experiment? Rethinking Political Ecology for the Anthropocene' in G. Bridge, T. Perreault and J. McCarthy (eds), *The Routledge Handbook of Political Ecology*. London: Routledge, pp. 102–114.

Buller, H. (2015), Animal geographies II: Methods. *Progress in Human Geography*, 39(3), 374–384.

Büscher, B. (2022), The nonhuman turn: Critical reflections on alienation, entanglement and nature under capitalism. *Dialogues in Human Geography*, 12(1), 54–73.

Chant, C. (2017), *Meet the Microbes*. London: Microbiology Society.

Clark, N. and Yusoff, K. (2017), Geosocial formations and the anthropocene. *Theory, Culture and Society*, 34(2–3), 3–23.

Davies, R. (2020), Physical distancing may be impossible on bus or train, DfT admits, *Guardian*, 12 May. Available at: www.theguardian.com/uk-news/2020/may/12/physical-distancing-public-transport-dft-government-advice-lockdown

Department of Health and Social Care. (2021), *Hands. Face. Space. Ventilation.* (video). Available at: www.youtube.com/watch?v=qYZMOG2kUWg (accessed 23 January 2023).

Dowling, R., Lloyd, K. and Suchet-Pearson, S. (2017), Qualitative methods II: 'More-than-human' methodologies and/in praxis. *Progress in Human Geography*, 41(6), 823–831.

Evans, J. and Lorimer, J. (2021), Taste-shaping-natures: Making novel miso with charismatic microbes and New Nordic fermenters in Copenhagen. *Current Anthropology*, 62(24), 361–375.

Garrett, B. L. (2011), Videographic geographies: Using digital video for geographic research. *Progress in Human Geography*, 35(4), 521–541.

Gillespie, K. and Collard, R., eds. (2015), *Critical Animal Geographies: Politics, Intersections and Hierarchies in a Multispecies World*. London: Routledge.

Greco, E. (2022), Engaging with the non-human turn: A response to Büscher. *Dialogues in Human Geography*, 12(1), 20438206221075704.

Greenhough, B. (2014), 'More-than-Human Geographies' in R. Lee et al. (eds), *The SAGE Handbook of Human Geography*. Los Angeles, London, New Delhi, Singapore and Washington, DC: SAGE, pp. 94–119.

Greenhough, B., Read, C. J., Lorimer, J., et al. (2020), Setting the agenda for social science research on the human microbiome. *Palgrave Communications*, 6(1), 1–11.

Gregg, M. and Seigworth, G. J., eds. (2010), *The Affect Theory Reader*. Durham, NC: Duke University Press.

Haraway, D. (2008) *When Species Meet*. Minneapolis, MN: University of Minnesota Press.

Haraway, D. (2016) *Staying with the Trouble: Making Kin in the Chthulucene*. Durham, NC: Duke University Press.

Hinchliffe, S., Kearnes, M. B., Degen, M., et al. (2005), Urban wild things: A cosmopolitical experiment. *Environment and Planning D: Society and Space*, 23(5), 643–658.

Hinchliffe, S. and Bingham, N. (2008), Securing life: The emerging practices of biosecurity. *Environment and Planning A*, 40(7), 1534–1551.

Hinchliffe, S. and Whatmore, S. (2017), 'Living Cities: Towards a Politics of Conviviality' in K. Anderson and B. Braun (eds), Environment. London: Routledge, pp. 555–570.

Hinchliffe, S., Butcher, A. and Rahman, M. M. (2018), The AMR problem: Demanding economies, biological margins, and co-producing alternative strategies. *Palgrave Communications*, 4(1), 1–12.

Hodgetts, T. and Lorimer, J. (2015), Methodologies for animals' geographies: Cultures, communication and genomics. *Cultural Geographies*, 22(2), 285–295.

Hughes, A., Roe, E. and Hocknell, S. (2021), Food supply chains and the antimicrobial resistance challenge: On the framing, accomplishments and limitations of corporate responsibility. *Environment and Planning A: Economy and Space*, 53(6), 1373–1390.

Hurley, P., and Turp, J. (2016), *In Our Hands* (video), featuring Michael Rosen's 'These are the Hands' poem. Available at: www.youtube.com/watch?v=W7xnaXSJab0&t=4s

Hutchinson, S. (2000), Waiting for the bus. *Social Text*, 18(2), 107–120.

Jacobs, J. (2013), Listen with your eyes: Towards a filmic geography. *Geography Compass*, 7(10), 714–728.

Jensen, O. (2009), Flows of meaning, cultures of movements: Urban mobility as meaningful everyday life practice. *Mobilities*, 4, 139–158

Kelley, L. (2016), *Bioart Kitchen: Art, Feminism and Technoscience*. London: Bloomsbury Publishing.

Latour, B. (1993), *The Pasteurization of France*. Cambridge, MA: Harvard University Press.

Little, P. (2020), Germ Defence. Available at: www.germdefence.org

Lorimer, J. (2010), Elephants as companion species: The lively biogeographies of Asian elephant conservation in Sri Lanka. *Transactions of the Institute of British Geographers*, 35(4), 491–506.

Lorimer, J. (2017), Parasites, ghosts and mutualists: A relational geography of microbes for global health. *Transactions of the Institute of British Geographers*, 42(4), 544–558.

Lorimer, J., Hodgetts, T., Grenyer, R., et al. (2019), Making the microbiome public: Participatory experiments with DNA sequencing in domestic kitchens. *Transactions of the Institute of British Geographers*, 44(3), 524–541.

Lynteris, C. (2020), *Human Extinction and the Pandemic Imaginary*. Abingdon and New York: Taylor & Francis.

Macduff, C., Macdonald, A. and Tsattalios, K. (2017), Unlocking the potential of visualisation approaches to address healthcare associated infections: A new international, cross-disciplinary, network. *Infection, Disease & Health*, 22, 19–20.

Mather, C. and Marshall, A. (2011), Biosecurity's unruly spaces. *The Geographical Journal*, 177(4), 300–310.

Menon, A. and Karthik, M. (2017), Beyond human exceptionalism: Political ecology and the non-human world. *Geoforum*, 79, 90–92.

Mitchell, R. E. (2015), *Bioart and the Vitality of Media*. Seattle, WA: University of Washington Press.

Public Health England. (2020a), *Beyond the Data: Understanding the Impact of COVID-19 on BAME Groups*. Public Health England. Available at: https://assets.publishing.service.gov.uk/government/uploads/system/uploads/attachment_data/file/892376/COVID_stakeholder_engagement_synthesis_beyond_the_data.pdf

Public Health England. (2020b), *Coronavirus Door Handle BSL* (video), 17 March . Available at: www.youtube.com/watch?v=bpyQJJGwe9k

Richardson-Ngwenya, P. (2014), Performing a more-than-human material imagination during fieldwork: Muddy boots, diarizing and putting vitalism on video. *Cultural Geographies*, 21(2), 293–299.

Roe, E. and Buser, M. (2016), Becoming ecological citizens: Connecting people through performance art, food matter and practices. *Cultural Geographies*, 23(4), 581–598.

Roe, E., Veal, C. and Hurley, P. (2019), Mapping microbial stories: Creative microbial aesthetic and cross-disciplinary intervention in understanding nurses' infection prevention practices. *Geo: Geography and Environment*, 6(1), e00076.

Roe, E., Veal, C., Hurley, P., et al. (2021), *Understanding Microbial Landscapes of the Bus during the Covid-19 Pandemic: December-2021 Report*. Available at: https://eprints.ncl.ac.uk/file_store/production/279182/25E56BC5-2EDC-4F9D-830A-4B86F10D9370.pdf

Sayaqle, M. (2020), *Impact of COVID-19 on Somali Community in Bristol*. Bristol Somali Youth Voice/Bristol Somali Forum. Available at: www.bristolhealthpartners.org.uk/uploads/documents/2020-11-30/1606743534-report-2020-impact-of-covid-19-on-somali-community-in-bristol.pdf

Shaker, R. (2021), 'Saying nothing is saying something': Affective encounters with the Muslim other in Amsterdam public transport. *Annals of the American Association of Geographers*, 111(7), 2130–2148.

Stengers, I. (1997), *Power and Invention: Situating Science*. Minneapolis, MN: University of Minnesota Press.

Swanson, H. (2017), Methods for multispecies anthropology: Thinking with salmon otoliths and scales. *Social Analysis*, 61(2), 81–99.

Taylor, A. and Pacini-Ketchabaw, V. (2018), *The Common Worlds of Children and Animals: Relational Ethics for Entangled Lives*. Abingdon and New York: Routledge.

TfL. (2012), *Understanding the Travel Needs of London's Diverse Communities*. Available at: https://content.tfl.gov.uk/BAME.pdf

Timmis, K., Cavicchioli, R., Garcia, J., et al. (2019), The urgent need for microbiology literacy in society. *Environmental Microbiology*, 21(5), 1513–1528.

Vasudevan, R. (2014), Biofilms: Microbial cities of scientific significance. *Journal of Microbiology and Experimentation*, 1(3), 84–98.

Veal, C. and Hawkins, H. (2020), 'Doing creative geographies: Exploring challenges and fulfilling promises' in A. de Dios and L. Kong (eds), *Handbook of the Geographies of Creativity*. Cheltenham, UK: Elgar Handbooks, pp. 352–369.

Waylen, G. (2021), How hypermasculine leadership may have affected early Covid-19 policy responses, LSE British Politics and Policy. Available at: https://blogs.lse.ac.uk/politicsandpolicy/hypermasculine-leadership/

Whatmore, S. (2006), Materialist returns: Practising cultural geography in and for a more-than-human world. *Cultural Geographies*, 13(4), 600–609.

Whatmore, S. (2017), 'Hybrid Geographies: Rethinking the 'Human' in Human Geography' in K. Anderson and B. Braun (eds), *Environment*. London: Routledge, pp. 411–428.

Wilson, H. (2011), Passing propinquities in the multicultural city: The everyday encounters of bus passengering. *Environment and Planning A*, 43(3), 634–649.

Wolfe, C. (2010), *What Is Posthumanism?* Minneapolis, MN: University of Minnesota Press.

2

Deafblindness, touch and COVID-19

Azadeh Emadi

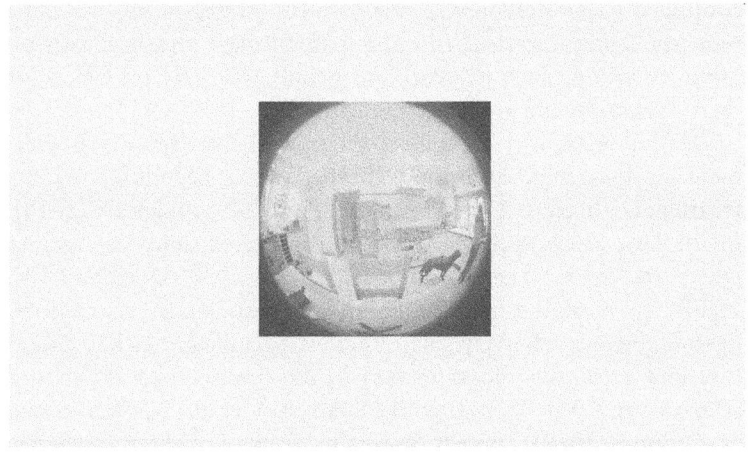

Figure 2.1 Still from VR video (Altered Perception Exhibition, 2022): Issy in her kitchen arranging flowers. All rights reserved.

In-depth understanding of deafblind people's perception and experiences of touch has become even more important due to the coronavirus (COVID-19) and subsequent wariness around touch and social distancing. At the end of March 2020, a laboratory study showed that COVID-19 could stay on plastic and stainless-steel surfaces for days. The study affirmed earlier guidelines by the World Health Organization (WHO) that the virus can be spread through touching contaminated surfaces (Lewis, 2021).[1] As a result, health agencies around the world, including the UK's National Health Service (NHS), advised people to frequently wash their hands and disinfect surfaces to help stop the spread of COVID-19.[2] As scientific studies grew, their understanding of touch as the primary form of transmission changed to transmission through droplets and particles that spread in the air from breathing and behaviours like talking or coughing (Van Doremalen et al., 2020). New preventive measures were introduced, such as 2-metre social distancing and meeting people only outside or in well-ventilated spaces. Nevertheless, this newer finding did not rule out the earlier claims about risks associated with touch or the emphasis on protocols of using hand sanitiser and decontaminating surfaces. Preventive measures such as disinfection, social distancing and wearing masks continued to be practised as main safety strategies. At the same time, the studies overlooked the impact of these measurements on minority groups such as deafblind people who rely on touch for their day-to-day life and communication.

Deafblindness is a complex condition of dual sensory impairment or loss that, according to the World Federation of the Deafblind, affects 0.2 per cent of the global population (2018). In the UK, nearly 400,000 people are affected, and the number is expected to increase beyond 600,000 by 2030 (Deafblind UK, 2020). Because the percentage of the population affected by deafblindness is relatively small, there is a significant lack of literature and social awareness related to the community's experience (Dammeyer, 2014; Jaiswal et al., 2018; Roy et al., 2018; Simcock and Wittich, 2019). There is especially a lack of qualitative enquiry into deafblind people's experiences (Jaiswal et al., 2018; World Federation of the Deafblind, 2018). Due to the lack of suitable awareness, the specific needs of deafblind people were missed from the safety measures and government policies introduced during the coronavirus pandemic. The project that led to this chapter, Touch Post-COVID-19, addressed this gap by gathering and studying the personal stories and experiences of the deafblind community across the UK during the pandemic. This project grew out of earlier research from 2019 that intended to understand sensory perception and explore deafblindness from the intersection of art, technology and culture. With the occurrence of COVID-19, the project turned its attention to the impact of the pandemic on the community, to question and explore impacts of touch deprivation on deafblind people's experiences during the pandemic.

To understand deafblind experiences, this interdisciplinary and public-facing research focused on audio diaries and video interviews, adopting Grounded Theory (GT) as a method for the collection and analysis of these data. Grounded Theory is concerned with a theory or concept that emerges from the systematic process of gathering and analysing data (Glaser and Strauss, 1968). A key position of GT is the way in which research remains purposefully open to the potential of gathered data in the research process. Anything that can help researchers generate concepts can be data, including an informal conversation, a text or image in the news, or a relevant object. For this research project, GT provided a framework for gathering and understanding data in relation to emerging themes and concepts. The research team worked with six members of the deafblind community from Scotland and England (identified and selected through the Deafblind Scotland and Deafblind UK organisations) and with various levels of impairment (from zero to partial hearing and seeing) and of different ages and genders. Researchers documented participants' experiences in the form of audio diaries and video interviews over 18 months beginning in November 2020. Audio diaries were the primary form of data in which participants' experiences and reflections were continuously gathered and analysed for common themes, issues or ideas that, in turn, informed the research direction. Over a 2-week period, participants were asked to record a diary, between 2 and 10 minutes long, describing their day-to-day experiences of touch, reflecting on their feelings, different events, interactions and physical and/or spatial encounters during the pandemic.[3] This process was repeated approximately every 4 months, per participant, over a total of 18 months (i.e., each participant recorded a 2-week continuous diary three times in total). After each stage, gathered data were studied and categorised according to the themes that occurred to the research team or resurfaced from the data (e.g., touching/scanning through feet, imagination as seeing, sensing nature, space) or identified issues (e.g., social distancing, discrimination, danger and vulnerability, hygiene). A one-to-one interview with participants followed each data collection and analysis stage.[4] From the identified themes and stories, open-ended questions were developed. Interviews aimed for an in-depth understanding of, for example, the impact of social distancing on participants' everyday activities; ways in which touch deprivation distorted their ability to map and memorise their everyday public spaces; and how enforced isolation increased their sense of dependency and vulnerability. The research team then designed a series of workshops with participants to explore emerging ideas and test possible solutions to identified challenges. The key aspect of our research method was the placement of participants at the centre of the research process through data collection, close conversations and researchers' involvement with participants. This close working together and use of audio diaries as the core of the method allowed researchers to identify the needs for and development of various outcomes such as new haptic technology; a policy brief and case study; art exhibitions and awareness-making workshops (to bring members of the deafblind community into dialogue with others from broader society); and co-creation of short films with selected participants about their experiences and stories.

This chapter highlights three stories from members of the deafblind community in Scotland and England, with a particular focus on one member for the sake of clarity.[5] The stories focus on touch as a 'visual' cue that offers spatial awareness, but is distorted due to imposed wariness about touch because of the pandemic. It is evident that for blind individuals, touch is crucial for spatial understanding and navigating the world (Alary et al., 2009; Goldreich and Kanics, 2003; Papadopoulos et al., 2012; Papagno et al., 2016). 'Visual mental imagery', an internal representation and recalling of objects and events unfolding in the 'visual' world, is significant for human understanding and identification of explicit shapes, spatial relations, memory formation and human behaviour (Borst et al., 2012). In sighted individuals, visual perception, the dominant sensory modality, usually precedes visual mental imagery and allows for successful spatial navigation and social connection. If a sighted person's physical ability to 'see' were to be reduced or diminished, they would have to develop different modes of understanding the nature of space and of social behaviour within it (Måseide and Grøttland, 2015). Because perception is made up of unified multisensory experiences, the absence or impairment of two senses has an even greater impact on deafblind individuals, making touch the main sensory modality that governs their understanding of the world (Department of Health, 1997; Jaiswal et al., 2018). During COVID-19, governments did not recognise how the deafblind population processes information and failed to consider them in their decision-making. Touch deprivation, caused by rules such as 2-metre social distancing and the individual's wariness towards touch, has disturbed their information processing and everyday activities. Consequently, the lack of considerate measures to include those with multisensory impairments pushed deafblind people into further isolation when this group is routinely excluded from society under normal circumstances.

2 metres distance: reaching towards

> As someone who is severely deaf and completely blind, I felt overnight I had lost a third sense, my sense of touch. To make matters worse, people around me faded away – voices had become so quiet that there was an eerie mumbling soundlessness all around. Nothing was making sense any more (Issy).

One of our research participants, Issy, has type II Usher Syndrome.[6] She lost her sight over time as an adult. Despite being completely blind and severely deaf, Issy has a passion for music and plays the flute often. Walking and swimming are her other regular activities. Imagination plays a significant role in her day-to-day experiences. In her audio diaries, she repeatedly refers to her perception as an 'inner eye'. With her 'inner eye', Issy noted, she catches things beyond the grasp of sight – like the almost solid nature of the winter air in the morning, or the enchanting atmosphere of a frozen landscape. For her, touch is about knowing, feeling, imagining and communicating. However, the pandemic severely impacted her experiences. The 2-metre social distancing rule enforced early in the pandemic imposed limitations above those experienced by sighted people.[7] For example, obtaining necessities or making simple contact with other people became impossible. The 2-metre distance can be frightening for someone relying on close proximity and touch as their only way of sensing the world. In her audio diary, Issy speaks about her struggles:

> Two-metre social distancing felt like the world had turned its back on me. I couldn't hear anyone anymore, my husband had to relay what people were saying to me. Two metres was also too far for me to reach out and touch what was around me, yet it is through touch that I get a sense of what a person may be like.

In a society that privileges vision as the dominant sense for knowing and thinking about the world (Belova, 2006; Brook, 2002), vision is inevitably considered the primary sensory modality capable of protecting us at times of crises like COVID-19. A blanket approach of a 2metre distancing rule presumed a particular subject and caused significant inequality for a part of society already marginalised due to impairments depending on touch. How can a blind person follow at 2 metres distance or know if others are keeping at a safe distance? In sighted people, eyes are directional and provide a safe distance from the perceived subject, making it possible for the brain to identify objects and events swiftly, assign meaning and respond accordingly without any unnecessary physical entanglements. This capacity to separate the perceiver from the perceived, driven by vision, permits spatial awareness based on what are known as 'allocentric' and 'egocentric' representation. Allocentric representation, which is the understanding of the position of items in space relative to each other and independent from the subject's orientation (object-centred) (Colombo et al., 2017), relies on distanced vision and is vital for long-term memory and navigation (Papadopoulos et al., 2012). On the other hand, egocentric spatial representation is about the position of objects in relation to the viewer (body-centred) – an example could be to say that the screen is in front of 'me'. For blind people, an awareness of egocentric referencing is significant for the development of strategies based on touch (haptic) that help them to extract information (coding) from near spaces and interpret that information to form meaning (representation). Haptic exploration of space (i.e., exploring space using touch) positions the body, not the eye, as a reference to encode the distance and orientation of objects (Papadopoulos et al., 2012; Postma et al., 2007).

Both allocentric and egocentric representations are repeatedly discussed in neuroscience and human biology literatures for their importance in creating visual mental imagery central to spatial memorisation (examples are Chen and Crawford, 2020; Colombo et al., 2017; Goldreich and Kanics, 2003). The role of what is formally called haptic egocentric referencing (locating objects according to one's own body position) in creating mental imagery and in navigation is less discussed in relation to sighted people because sight tends to overshadow the role of touch and haptic engagement in forming mental images, even though egocentric referencing stays relevant. However, in the case of a deafblind person's awareness, haptic egocentric representation cannot be replaced by other sense modalities. For Issy, spatial memorisation through haptic egocentric referencing is the only way to construct a mental image of her surrounding:

> If I go out, I don't walk through air; if I do walk through air, I will be disoriented. I have got to go and touch a wall. As soon as I touch the wall my mind sees a wall. A wall in my head, is just opened up. It is almost you reach and touch, and is magic..., it is in your head. It materialises.

Constructing a mental image through a haptic encounter requires its own pace. Unlike sighted people, blind individuals perceive and traverse the space slowly as they '[investigate] tactile and auditory qualities' of a site. This 'corporeal, searching, and step-wise experience of space' is more detailed and consequently requires more attention and time (Måseide and Grøttland, 2015: 596–597). For deafblind people, hearing loss/impairment is an added challenge that makes touch the primary mode of perception. Issy and other research participants expressed this continuous tactile scanning of the space as laborious and exhausting because the body is always in a 'state of alertness'. Understandably, sighted people often attempt to remove obstacles for a blind person or pre-empt their motivation and hand them what they think a blind person might be 'looking for' or 'scanning for'.[8] However, what to a sighted person is an 'obstacle', to a deafblind individual can be a 'pile of information' necessary for their imagination and spatial awareness. By clearing their path without fully considering their different mode of perception, sighted people erase necessary information and sensations from their world. This consequently makes spaces difficult to navigate and unsafe because, as Issy says, in an open space, 'there is nothing to relate to'.

Social distancing, placed as a safety measure during COVID-19, did not consider these other perceptual modes and consequently took away the necessary haptic references from deafblind people. This enforced open space distorted participants' spatial awareness and ability to form mental images. Issy highlights that instead of safety, it brought anxiety: '[With] two-metre distance, I lost all forms of communications. This is a form of discrimination, putting distance between me and my life.' For our participants, their vital mode of experiencing and communicating with the world was taken away under the banner of care and protection. At the same time, other people could still go on with their lives (even if restricted). To people like Issy, this felt like a one-sided approach to the pandemic that disregarded their presence in society. It can be argued that the deafblind community were already invisible and excluded from decision-making, and COVID-19 has only shed light on pre-existing inequalities. For our participants, simple tasks like moving around in public spaces, shopping in a supermarket or taking public transport were not an option anymore, and their exacerbated isolation continued beyond the early stage of the pandemic; as Issy says:

> [T]he world both passed me by and left me constantly conflicted: Do I allow people into my space so that I can interact and make sense of the world, risking catching the virus, or do I ask people to respect the two-metre social distance rule and allow a creeping sense of isolation to overwhelm my emotional wellbeing?[9]

For our participants, this convoluted emotion was an added toll on anxieties associated with the pandemic.

Distorted: scanning through feet

COVID-19 distorted participants' ability to form mental maps of spaces as well as their already existing images. For a moment, imagine that one morning you step out of your home only to discover that your neighbourhood and familiar streets are suddenly and completely different. You may feel confused, anxious and unsure about how to get to your destination, continuously losing orientation and getting lost. Now, imagine it happening to you every other day, if not every day. This was Issy's experience as she attempted a daily walk in her familiar neighbourhood after the easing of the lockdown and the phased re-opening of hospitalities.[10] Cafés and restaurants were expanding outside and changing pedestrian areas every day. In her walk, Issy continuously bumped into 'unexpected' obstacles that distorted her mental image of the neighbourhood. She experienced great anxiety to the point of becoming tearful in the middle of the street and decided to take refuge in her house and rely on close family members when going out. The pandemic even impacted her steps and the feeling of the ground under her feet.

When we think about touch, particularly in the context of blindness and communication, it is common to think of hands and fingertips. Roger, another participant, highlights that 'touch uses all aspects of the body – from the top of the head to feel the sunlight, to the feet, which are important for feeling where you are on the street … Feet are important for feeling'. All our participants highlighted the prominence to their perception of touching through their feet. Yet the importance of feet as a form of touch is largely overlooked.

The placement of the eyes on the head gives a sighted person an immediate awareness of the front field that allows for visually orienting themselves. For a blind person, on the other hand, forward-oriented perception is based on haptic perception (Harris et al., 2015; Iachini et al., 2014) and assisted by hand touch and the use of a white-red cane (for a deafblind person). Even if they choose to focus on the front for their navigation, their perceptual field encompasses the whole body and its complete alertness, particularly while walking. Through their feet, they scan and perceive the environment and recognise characteristics and qualities of different spaces, such as the change of material structure and texture or the shift on the edge of a pavement. This continuous touching and scanning of the ground beneath their feet, in addition to identifying objects in the space through hand touch or cane, is significant for effectively encoding the space to form a mental map.

However, COVID-19 restricted participants' ability to touch through hands and feet, causing them distress and anxiety and interfering with their effort to create a mental map that made them feel safe and more independent. John, another research participant, explains scanning via feet as part of a 'holistic way' of feeling through the body and gathering various fragmented pieces of information from his surroundings. He describes combining these fragmented pieces of information to create a mental image, like solving a jigsaw puzzle.

John has been severely deaf from birth and now has 5 per cent vision left. Like other participants, he cannot immediately know the space beyond his proximity. It requires a laborious and time-consuming process of touching, feeling, evaluating and interpreting one element before moving to the next one. John describes this process as exhausting, with 'a lot of concentration and making up pictures', but necessary for creating a mental map of space in relation to his body. 'When you think back, you think: how did I do that [distinguishing between different rooms without the help of vision] but it's more down to a holistic way of feeling. You know your body, your feet, your nose, etc.' Once a mental image of a site is created from repeated scanning through touch, John can navigate through that space more efficiently and independently because he is now aware of the spatial configuration of items in the place independent from his body (excluding the moving objects and people). 'If someone is blind or visually impaired or whatever – they are often very, very conscious of their space, and they know where things are. And the worst thing you can do is move something in that space.'

In addition to the challenges of social distancing for our deafblind participants, this continuous shifting and reconfiguring of public spaces disturbed their ability to map space and navigate it.

Reconciliation: joy or fear of touch

Emergency measures introduced during crises often tend to change social norms and reshape human behaviours (Brailsford, 2014; Gross and Ní Aoláin, 2006; Nohrstedt and Weible, 2010; Taplin, 1971). Social distancing and isolation are no exception. Even after easing these measures, their ongoing negative impact was evident in the gathered data. 'Even now, with the relaxing of social distancing, the joy I had in reaching out to touch and link arms with other people has become subdued and cautious, as I warily navigate my world through my hands and my sense of touch', says Issy. An ongoing sense of isolation and fear of touch affected our participants' daily activities and limited their already minimal social interactions. The audio diaries and many conversations with deafblind individuals indicate that 'reminding' sighted people or 'consciously utilising' their other sense modalities for perceiving can assist in counteracting the negative impact of the pandemic, such as further isolation and social exclusion of the deafblind community. Building shared spaces of interaction and communication into the fabric of society is essential for an inclusive culture and a sensible body politic conscientious of other bodies.

Neuroscientists and psychologists have largely argued that our perception of events and objects comes from the integration of different types of information received from all our senses (see Baumard and Osiurak, 2019; Betti et al., 2021; Dehaene and Changeux, 2011; Faivre et al., 2017; Mudrik et al., 2014). The holistic experience of the senses and the process of meaning-making results from the vortex of all sensory inputs, giving us an understanding of the world as it is known. We also know that information processing is central to making sense of the world and distinguishing between the self and others. The cultural theorist, Erin Manning, argues that the body is not static as a receiver, but active; '[to] sense is not to simply receive input – it is to invent' (2009: 212). The body does not hold on to the information. Instead, information in-forms a new relation with whatever the body has encountered, originating movement and change. Perception in all modes always involves this reciprocal relationship of reception and action. But touch that is in implicit interaction with other senses and the force of reaching towards the other puts the body in motion, both the 'sensing body' and the 'political body' (Manning, 2007). Bodies of all forms and colours touch and are touched by their surroundings, affected in each encounter. Touch as reaching towards is an act that draws 'other[s] into relation' (Manning, 2007: 15). These relations are not free of risk. Unlike 'looking', which involves a safe distance, touch connotes an entanglement that beholds danger – one is affected as much as affecting the other. Early in the pandemic, realising that 'my' touch equally threatens 'me' and 'others' brought many conversations on our interconnectedness. However, as Manning points out, touch is not only physical but can be psychological, cultural and political, with bodies potentially changing each other in exchanges taking place through each interaction. Starting from how the body, a single unit, processes information and initiates movement, she magnifies the role of bodies as the nexus of shape-shifting larger estates. She argues that there are bodies in motion that resist the predefinition of subjectivity. They continuously set in motion the world around them – the body not confirming and thus challenging the collective perception. For Manning, how we define the body forms our politics. While questioning the dualistic mind–body/reason–senses model, Manning explores the sensing body to challenge existing state-centred political structures that lack flexibility. The existence of 'unstable bodies', which she refers to as 'the other, the outside, the homeless, the refugee or the stranger, the sexual "deviant"' challenge the fixity of the politic (2007: 95). These bodies, continuously re-inventing themselves, can unrest normative bodies that represent the social image as a whole. In 'relational' environments, bodies continuously learn from and build alongside other bodies and can shape-shift the whole for a more inclusive society.

Conclusion

My own very first meeting with a deafblind person before the pandemic was perplexing because I had no previous experience of communicating with deafblind people. It was the holding of hands to communicate and sit together that moved me and my thoughts. It triggered a mode of knowing the 'other' that is not rational but, at that moment, meant simply accepting the other body and responding to it by observing your senses entangling with the other. Our participants unanimously expressed a great desire and need for public awareness of how they interacted with space, as well as for varying sensory technologies and experiences that would help them be part of the larger society.

Roger describes discovering new relations through touch while expressing the impact of the pandemic on his daily activities. For Roger, touching is more than receiving sensory input or holding on to information. It is a chance for a new perceptual experience and to form a new 'relation'. Corneal scars and glaucoma suffered during childhood limit what Roger can perceive quite a bit – he is able to see colour, but with little definition. Trees, one of his favourite things, appear as a golden or green mass. When gardening, he 'observes' plants and trees: he can 'feel' the seasons, and the maturing of plants and branches, through the bendability, texture and direction of the growth. Roger says there is a 'magic' to touch – 'you can feel the energy of things'. He describes it as a joy and energy that, like inhaling air, expands his perceptual experience. But the pandemic transformed his joyful experience of touch into a feeling of threat to his safety. He couldn't hold people's arms anymore and, even with hearing aids, communication was not easy. Simple everyday tasks became significantly challenging:

> Meeting friends when walking out has become a real challenge. I need to be close and in a fairly quiet environment to hear and for years, I have had a particular difficulty recognising the voice of those I actually know well. The COVID-19 mask makes it all much worse...

With the relaxing of restrictions, Roger began going places again. But without knowing his distance from others or being able to assess the safety of his environment, he had no option but to stay mostly passive for other people to act first, like someone squeezing his arm:

> I have never really known when it is my turn to speak to an assistant at the counter –and when there are two masks and a screen between us ... not much hope in that situation. The worst episode of this kind occurred on my first visit back to our local café, which we love. I only wanted a coffee and cake, and I should have written out my order for her on my phone, but that's not easy either for a blind chap... So having failed to communicate with each other, a nearby child screamed and I flipped and tried to leave. Taking pity on me, the assistant came round from behind the counter, and we were able to agree a deal. When it came to me paying, the machine had a touch screen, no physical buttons so I could not use it. She squeezed my arm, very nice, and told me it was on the house, lovely coffee and carrot cake.

A simple gesture of touch communication that was considered risky earlier offered Roger compassion, safety and comfort. Roger is eager to let sighted people know that touch is not always about making up for lack of vision. Deafblind people's tactile world contains much joy. He brings us back to the importance of touch as a mode of communication based on felt knowledge. Even though our body does not distil its sensation to one sensory organ (such as the eyes), the perceptual and epistemological ranking of vision over other senses has largely overlooked other experiential modes of knowing. We may argue that physiologically, it is common for most people's awareness to be occupied by a dominant sense that overrides overall sensory experiences. Therefore, a sighted person may not easily experience the joy in Roger's tactile world or the extent to which social distancing has impacted Issy's 'inner eye'. Yet, the interwoven nature of sensory experience can offer various modes of knowing. Following Manning's description, information processing is as much about apprehension and setting relations as about distinguishing between self and others (2009). When explored fully, the joy in a deafblind person's tactile world offers a way of seeing and hearing that, instead of being grounded on distance, is based on intimate and interconnected ways of knowing. Here, the 'joy' is not about sensory stimulation but a close encounter that brings about comprehension and connection in the form of a slowed contemplative observation not overshadowed by one or two senses.

The pandemic has exposed and exacerbated pre-existing inequalities in our society. The gathered data and stories from our participants highlighted the fact that restrictions had impacted them unproportionately. The 2-metres social distancing had the most notable negative impact. It took away their primary means of communication to reach out, feel the world and be part of society. As a result, access to shops such as supermarkets, and consequently to food, was compromised, mainly when online shopping was not an option due to their disability or if it involved touch-screen payments. They found it impossible to navigate public spaces without feeling distressed and powerless, when they could not know whether distancing rules were breached, and more so because of their dependency on close proximity and touch for navigation and communication. Restaurants and bars expanding into public spaces, and shifting the layout of pedestrian sites, added another layer of challenge and distorted participants' mental image of their neighbouring sites. Touch, which initially was presented as the main form of transmission of the coronavirus, continued to be perceived as the main hazard, even though later scientific findings focused on airborne particles. In the absence of proper and targeted communication from the government, our participants followed self-imposed limitations, such as avoiding touching surfaces despite their dependency on touch. Due to a blanket approach to safety measures that were introduced, our participants were pushed into further isolation and exclusion from society, with increased dependency on family and friends for support. They were more likely to feel lonely, anxious and frightened, expressing deep disappointment that their lives and needs seemed invisible to the decision-makers.

If we are to build a fairer, more inclusive society for the deafblind community, we need to remove the existing barriers and learn from them about their perception and needs. One way is to utilise new sensory modalities (e.g., with haptic technologies – see Kassem et al., 2022) and create environments that enrich diverse modes of experiences and communications. Deafblindness needs to be more central to our understanding of different perceptual experiences. Touch, as a concept that evokes interwoven relations and knowledge, can help us to re-evaluate some of the existing socio-environmental settings and approaches that pre-empt what a group of people may need or experience. The joy in deafblind people's touch teaches us about the 'thinking' (as contemplating and expanding one's perception) that happens only in a close encounter.

Acknowledgements

This research was approved by the University of Glasgow ethics approval committee. Informed consent was obtained from all subjects involved in the study. The author acknowledges financial support from the UK Arts and Humanities Research Council (AHRC) within the UK Research and Innovation (UKRI) Rapid Response to COVID-19 initiative (grant AH/V012797/1) and from the UK Engineering and Physical Sciences Research Council (grant EP/T00097X/1). The author acknowledges research partners, Deafblind Scotland and Deafblind UK, with particular recognition of the research participants.

Research team

Azadeh Emadi, Daniele Faccio, Mitch Miller, Annie Runkel, Piergiorgio Caramazza, Khaled Kassem

Notes

1 www.who.int/docs/default-source/coronaviruse/who-china-joint-mission-on-covid-19-final-report.pdf
2 www.nhs.uk/conditions/covid-19/how-to-avoid-catching-and-spreading-covid-19/

3 Participants were given a choice to either use their mobile phone or the provided SONY ICD-PX240 digital voice recorder. Their preference was their mobile phone because it was always with them. After every 2 weeks of recording, the gathered audio data would be sent to the research team. A guide communicator from Deafblind Scotland or Deafblind UK would collate and send the audio to the team if required.
4 During lockdowns, interviews took place via Zoom with the assistance of an interpreter from Deafblind Scotland when necessary. After the easing of restrictions, some of the interviews were in person.
5 These stories are also featured in an article for the Insights series of The Conversation (see Emadi, 2022).
6 Usher Syndrome II is an inherited condition that affects hearing and vision, often in the form of early hearing loss and progressive vision loss that usually starts in the teenage years.
7 The government imposed social distancing as a legal requirement to limit close contact with others during the coronavirus. Local Authorities and operators had to implement the social distancing guidelines and ensure they were followed. The rule required minimising time spent outside the home, keeping to 2 metres from anyone outside a person's own household, and using physical barriers or screens in certain public places.
8 It should be noted that it is equally not easy for a sighted person to turn his or her attention to the sense of touch as a way of knowing the world. For a sighted person, slowing down to sense through touch can also be challenging.
9 Although guide dogs, for those who have one, are a great help, they don't respond to social distancing, and they don't stop people from touching a deafblind person to grab their attention.
10 In the UK, people were first ordered to stay home on 23 March 2020. The government introduced the 2-metres social distancing rule and eased the lockdown on 23 June 2020, with pubs, restaurants and hairdressers re-opening on 4 July 2020. Since the easing of the lockdown on 23 June, the hospitality sector, where possible, has been using outside spaces to provide services to customers safely.

References

Alary, Flamine, Duquette, M., Goldstein, R., et al. (2009), Tactile acuity in the blind: A closer look reveals superiority over the sighted in some but not all cutaneous tasks. *Neuropsychologia*, 47(10), 2037–2043.

Baumard, Josselin and Osiurak, François (2019), Is bodily experience an epiphenomenon of multisensory integration and cognition?. *Frontiers in Human Neuroscience*, 13, 316.
Belova, Olga (2006), The event of seeing: A phenomenological perspective on visual sense-making. *Culture and Organization*, 12(2), 93–107.
Betti, Sonia, Castiello, Umberto and Begliomini, Chiara (2021), Reach-to-grasp: A multisensory experience. *Frontiers in Psychology*, 12, 614471.
Borst, Gregoire, Ganis, G., Thompson, W. L., et al. (2012), Representations in mental imagery and working memory: Evidence from different types of visual masks. *Memory & Cognition*, 40(2), 204–217.
Brailsford, Sally C. (2014), 'Modeling Human Behavior – An (Id)Entity Crisis?' in *Proceedings of the Winter Simulation Conference 2014*. IEEE. doi: 10.1109/WSC.2014.7020006
Brook, Isis (2002), Experiencing interiors: Oculacentrism and Merleau-Ponty's redeeming of the role of vision. *Journal of the British Society for Phenomenology*, 33(1), 68–77.
Chen, Ying and Crawford, J. Douglas (2020), Allocentric representations for target memory and reaching in human cortex. *Annals of the New York Academy of Sciences*, 1464(1), 142–155.
Colombo, Desirée, Serino, Silvia, Tuena, Cosimo, et al. (2017), Egocentric and allocentric spatial reference frames in aging: A systematic review. *Neuroscience and Biobehavioral Reviews*, 80, 605–621.
Dammeyer, Jesper (2014), Deafblindness: A review of the literature. *Scandinavian Journal of Public Health*, 42(7), 554–562.
Deafblind UK. (2020), What is deafblindness? Available at: https://deafblind.org.uk/get_support/what-is-deafblindness/ (accessed 10 March 2020).
Dehaene, Stanislas and Changeux, Jean-Pierre (2011), Experimental and theoretical approaches to conscious processing. *Neuron*, 70(2), 200–227.
Department of Health. (1997), *Think Dual Sensory: Good Practice Guidelines for Older People with Dual Sensory Loss*. London: The Stationery Office.
Emadi, Azadeh (2022), The magic of touch: How deafblind people taught us to 'see' the world differently during COVID. The Conversation, 10 October. Available at: https://theconversation.com/the-magic-of-touch-how-deafblind-people-taught-us-to-see-the-world-differently-during-covid-191698 (accessed 10 October 2022).
Faivre, Nathan, Arzi, Anat, Lunghi, Claudia, et al. (2017), Consciousness is more than meets the eye: A call for a multisensory study of subjective experience. *Neuroscience of Consciousness*, 1,nix003.
Glaser, Barney G. and Strauss, Anselm L. (1968), *The Discovery of Grounded Theory: Strategies for Qualitive Research*. London: Weidenfeld & Nicolson.
Goldreich, Daniel and Kanics, Ingrid M. (2003), Tactile acuity is enhanced in blindness. *The Journal of Neuroscience*, 23(8), 3439–3445.

Gross, Oren and Ní Aoláin, Fionnuala (2006), *Law in Times of Crisis: Emergency Powers in Theory and Practice*. Cambridge: Cambridge University Press.

Harris, Laurence R., Carnevale, M. J., D'Amour, S., et al. (2015), How our body influences our perception of the world. *Frontiers in Psychology*, 6, 87.

Iachini, Tina, Ruggiero, Gennaro and Ruotolo, Francesco (2014), Does blindness affect egocentric and allocentric frames of reference in small and large scale spaces? *Behavioural Brain Research*, 273, 73–81.

Jaiswal, Atul, Aldersey, Heather, Wittich, Walter, et al. (2018), Participation experiences of people with deafblindness or dual sensory loss: A scoping review of global deafblind literature. *PloS One*, 13(9), 1–26.

Kassem, Khaled, Caramazza, P., Mitchell, K. J., et al. (2022), Real-time scene monitoring for deaf-blind people. *Sensors*, 22(19). https://doi.org/10.3390/s22197136

Lewis, Dyani (2021), COVID-19 rarely spreads through surfaces. So why are we still deep cleaning? *Nature (London)*, 590(7844), 26–28.

Manning, Erin (2007), *Politics of Touch: Sense, Movement, Sovereignty*. Minneapolis, MN: University of Minnesota Press. doi: 10.5749/j.ctttsxrz

Manning, Erin (2009), Taking the next step: Touch as technique. *The Senses & Society*, 4(2), 211–225.

Måseide, Per and Grøttland, Håvar (2015), Enacting blind spaces and spatialities: A sociological study of blindness related to space, environment and interaction. *Symbolic Interaction*, 38(4), 594–610.

Mudrik, Liad, Faivre, Nathan and Koch, Christof (2014), Information integration without awareness. *Trends in Cognitive Sciences*, 18(9), 488–496.

Nohrstedt, Daniel and Weible, Christopher M. (2010) The logic of policy change after crisis: Proximity and subsystem interaction. *Risk, Hazards & Crisis in Public Policy*, 1(2), 1–32.

Papadopoulos, Konstantinos, Koustriava, Eleni and Kartasidou, Lefkothea (2012), Spatial coding of individuals with visual impairments. *The Journal of Special Education*, 46(3), 180–190.

Papagno, Costanza, Cecchetto, Carlo, Pisoni, Alberto, et al. (2016), Deaf, blind or deafblind: Is touch enhanced? *Experimental Brain Research*, 234(2), 627–636.

Postma, Albert, Zuidhoek, Sander, Noordzij, Matthijs L., et al. (2007), Differences between early-blind, late-blind, and blindfolded-sighted people in haptic spatial-configuration learning and resulting memory traces. *Perception*, 36(8), 1253–1265. doi:10.1068/p5441

Roy, Alana, McVilly, Keith R. and Crisp, Beth R. (2018), Preparing for inclusive consultation, research and policy development: Insights from the field of deafblindness. *Journal of Social Inclusion*, 9(1), 71.

Simcock, Peter and Wittich, Walter (2019), Are older deafblind people being left behind? A narrative review of literature on deafblindness through the lens of the United Nations Principles for Older People. *The Journal of Social Welfare & Family Law*, 41(3), 339–357.

Taplin, J. R. (1971), Crisis theory: Critique and reformulation. *Community Mental Health Journal*, 7(1), 13–23.
Van Doremalen, Neeltje, Bushmaker, Trenton, Morris, Dylan H., et al. (2020), Aerosol and surface stability of SARS-CoV-2 as compared with SARS-CoV-1. *The New England Journal of Medicine*, 382(16), 1564–1567.
World Federation of the Deafblind. (2018), *Initial Global Report on the Situation and Rights of Persons with Deafblindness*, International Disability Alliance. Available at: www.internationaldisabilityalliance.org/wfdb-global-report (accessed 10 January 2021).

3

Testing, testing: What about the instructions?

Sue Walker, Josefina Bravo and Al Edwards

Recent decades have seen the steady growth of clinical diagnostic tests that can be used at home, at pharmacies or general practitioner (GP) practices (St John and Price, 2014). From home pregnancy tests to Fitbits and smart watches, the analytical chemistry and analysis technology has been miniaturised and automated, allowing an increasing range of tests to be taken outside laboratories and hospitals, and brought into the community. Following the roll-out of regular home and workplace testing for COVID-19 during the pandemic, an initial dramatic scale-up of centralised testing was followed by widely publicised mass-testing. Following early pilots exploring the accuracy of rapid lateral flow tests (LFTs), the UK Government purchased and distributed tests into the community before publication (*BMJ*, 2021: 374 n1637). Educational testing was prioritised (in higher education from November 2020 and in schools from January 2021) and subsequently, rapid tests for home use were distributed freely; for example, from most community pharmacies by April 2021 (gov.uk, 2021).[1] To accompany the tests, different kinds of instructions explained to people how to carry out an LFT. These tests usually involve taking a sample from your nose and/or mouth, using a swab. The swab is then mixed with a solution and drops are put into a special device. The results are available in ten to 30 minutes depending on the kind of test. Instructions for these tests range from booklets that accompany National Health Service (NHS) and government testing kits, to videos, animations and posters produced by people of all ages from many different backgrounds and with different experiences. During the pandemic, many people learned how to carry out a test – and became proficient and confident about carrying it out accurately. In the near term, more use of lateral flow tests for community infections such as influenza can be expected. Many community testing services were established during the pandemic for remote monitoring, especially for managing long-term conditions. Many of these have been retained beyond the pandemic, as patients and clinicians alike prefer point-of-care testing to a return to slow and inconvenient hospital clinic visits. As more community testing takes place with new point-of-care tests, more and better instructions will be needed to ensure the tests are carried out safely and accurately.

This chapter intervenes in this landscape, through a study of the design and usability of instructions for point-of-use COVID-19 lateral flow rapid tests. At its heart is an argument that such tests don't simply need better instructions, but that we need a richer, more nuanced account of what is meant by 'good instructions' in the first place. We start by outlining the differences between 'instructions for use' and 'point-of-use' instructions and draw from existing design research to argue the benefits of simple instructions for point-of-use. After explaining our approach and summarising our methods, the focus turns to our exploration of design features to create effective point-of-use instructions. Although focused on current lateral flow rapid tests for COVID-19, the findings are applicable to any community-based testing technology and medical condition. In particular, we describe the development of a toolkit to support the creation of point-of-use instructions, taking account of views from diagnostic industry members to inform an understanding of how instructions are produced currently and what guidance might be helpful. The chapter outlines unresolved tensions between the needs of final users and the constraints posed by needing to meet regulations within timeframes. The benefits of user-friendly point-of-use instructions can be leveraged not only in home tests, but also in community testing settings, to be used by healthcare professionals as well as patients.

Why are instructions so critical for community diagnostic testing?

What makes these instructions for point-of-care diagnostic tests especially critical is the big jump between laboratory testing versus out-of-laboratory alternatives that adds significant pressure to the quality of these instructions (Figure 3.1). Laboratory testing is supervised and controlled by teams of highly trained staff, with a range of quality control and certification processes in place, and many laboratory tests have regular calibration or checking

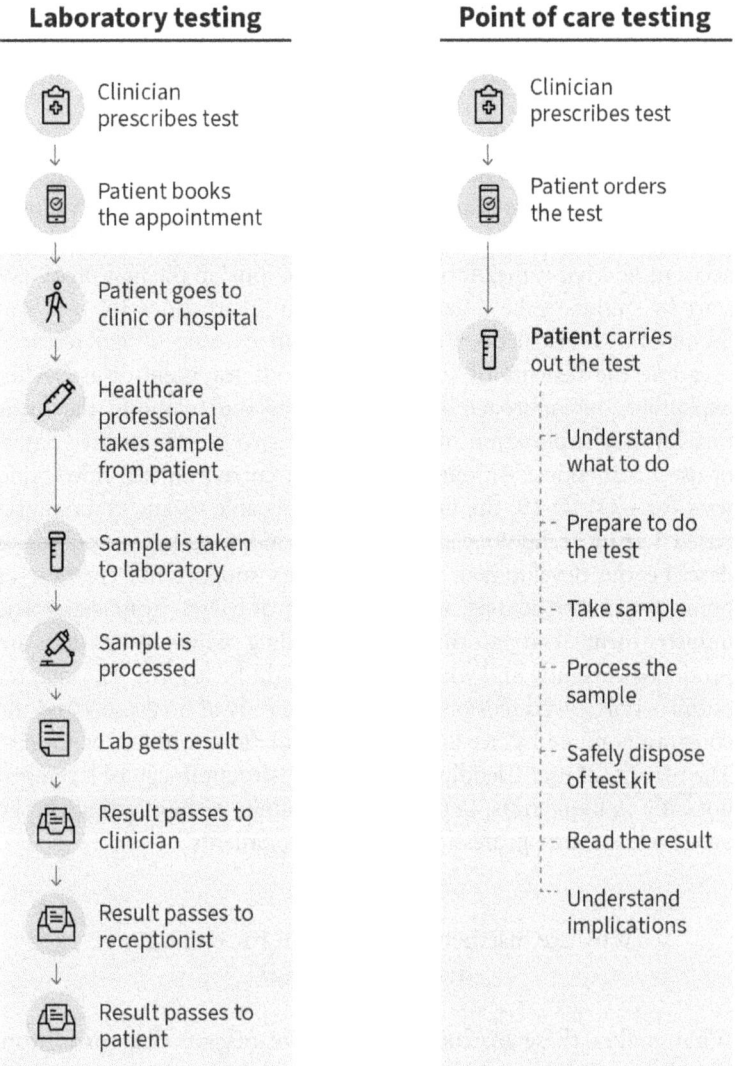

Figure 3.1 Laboratory testing versus point-of-care testing

processes to ensure that tests are operated correctly. The operation of such tests is less dependent on the clarity of instructions, and many more layers are in place to ensure results are accurate and the testing process is safe and effective. In contrast, home or community-based tests rely on non-trained users, often without any checking or training. This places great pressure on the quality of instructions to substitute for expert supervision.

Procedural instructions for diagnostic tests: an overview

All diagnostic tests have to include 'instructions for use' (IFUs), produced in line with a regulatory framework of principles that includes general guidance about the structure of information and its visual organisation (IEEE, IEC and ISO, 2019). This guidance for setting out instructions aligns with good practice, but tends to be applied with little consideration of the needs of final users, and the information is often embedded in a leaflet that contains other regulatory information (aimed at laboratories, expert users, or information required for liability reasons). Upon inspection, the graphic presentation of information and the different kinds of information contained in some IFUs suggest their role as documents for risk control and liability management, rather than vehicles of clear information designed to improve user experience. Figure 3.2 shows a typical IFU annotated to indicate the parts that challenge ease of use for lay first-time users. Cherne et al. (2020), who examined how healthcare professionals, patients and lay caregivers engaged with IFUs, included 'design elements' in their review. They found that bulleted lists, pictures and logical organisation engaged users, whereas too much text, small type and lack of clear structure to the information were thought to be off-putting. These observations support an established view that good information design can help by making sure that information is clearly structured and understood so that it can be acted upon (Dickinson and Gallina, 2017; Tong et al., 2014; Walker, 2017; Waller and VandenBerg, 2017).

Our research investigated the design and ease of use of instructions for carrying out COVID-19 LFTs at the point of use. Unlike the mandatory IFUs specified by regulations, point-of-use instructions take account of the needs of intended users and are

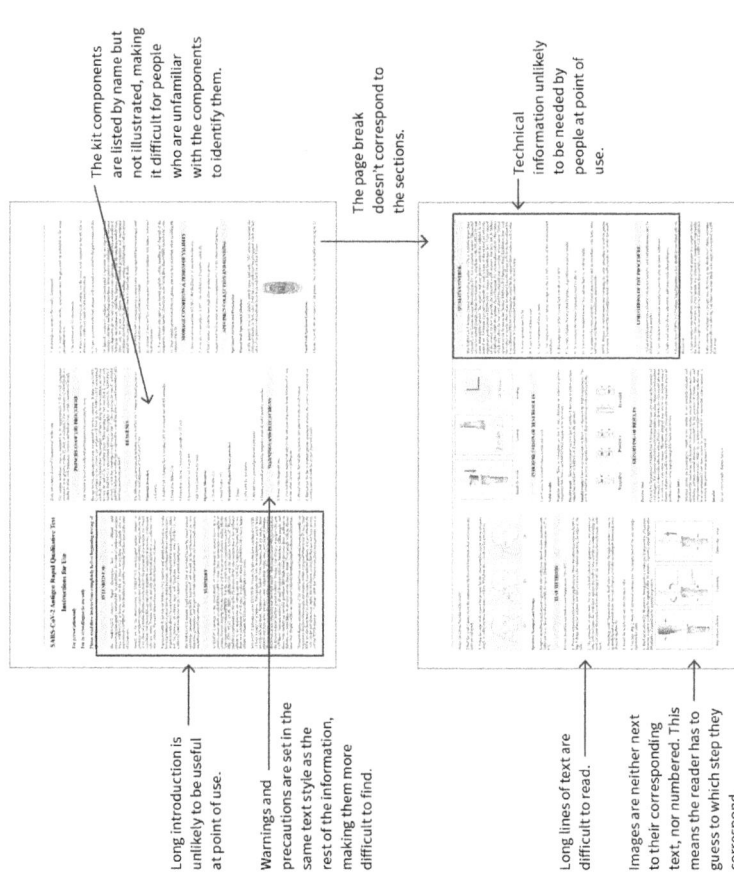

Figure 3.2 COVID-19 self-test

designed to be easy to read and follow. Design features that reduce the effort of readers include ensuring that there are clearly identified sections and procedural steps, the action steps are explained through words and pictures, and the text is easy to read. This is affirmed by observations from Atchison et al. (2020) who, in relation to instructions for COVID-19 tests, found that diagrams with clear visual cueing and simple language helped lay users, and Kierkegaard et al. (2021), who reviewed the quality of information supporting LFTs, and suggested that more attention should be paid to the information needs of lay users and context of use.

There is already considerable knowledge about how people use and interpret instructions, the types of information they need and best practice for the visual organisation of text and image.[2] We reviewed and applied this work as appropriate to explore the graphic presentation of parts of the test where mistakes were made and that then affected test accuracy and validity.

Information design approach and methods

The project, Information Design for Diagnostics: Ensuring Confidence and Accuracy for Home Sampling and Home Testing, combined information design research and practice with bioscience research. The project team included partners in the diagnostic testing industry and public health. The bioscientists brought understanding of the chemistry and working of the tests and, importantly, had a vision for the future relevance of community-based diagnostic testing. Information design research, in relation to health communication, as Walker has noted elsewhere (2019: 2), contributes by:

- considering the selection and presentation of the information provider's message in relation to the purposes, skills, experience, preferences and circumstances of the intended users;
- co-designing with information providers and intended users in the development of prototype solutions;
- finding out whether protypes in development or completed documents work for their intended audience and circumstances of use through qualitative and quantitative methods;
- offering creative solutions to the visual organisation of information through the treatment of the text and the design.[3]

We followed a process well established within information design of Discovery–Transforming–Making (Waller and VandenBerg, 2017), consisting of exploring the problem and identifying areas where the visual organisation of text and images may present difficulties for readers, developing a range of solutions, and, through evaluation, narrowing down to prototypes. Our project used a 'rapid design decision-making' process to identify and explore the design features that improve instructions for members of the public. Evidence from user research and existing best practice informed the design of a prototype for point-of-use instructions for a COVID-19 lateral flow test. Working with members of the in-vitro diagnostic testing industry, we applied our prototype to see how our approach could be transferred to other kinds of tests. Semi-structured interviews were conducted to gather industry members' views of the importance of instructions for use, and to better understand the applications of a design toolkit. These stages of the projects are covered in the following sections.

Prototype development: rapid design decision-making

In a previous study with low-cost 3-D printed home-testing kits, bioscience members of the research team had found that when they carried out tests with users to check ease of use, instructions for using the kit they provided needed improvement (Needs et al., 2020). They identified the parts of the test that needed to be carried out correctly to ensure accurate test results. For the purposes of this project, we were therefore able to narrow down the variables we could realistically evaluate given our time constraints. Areas that appeared to cause problems were procedural steps that included actions such as 'squeeze' and 'rotate', that are difficult to describe in words and pictures; putting the correct number of drops in the test device; and interpreting the results. This work informed the focus of the design approach, which used a range of techniques to enable rapid design decision-making. This comprised a review and distillation of existing research, stakeholder engagement and application of tacit information design knowledge (as two members of the research team were practising designers) (Figure 3.3).

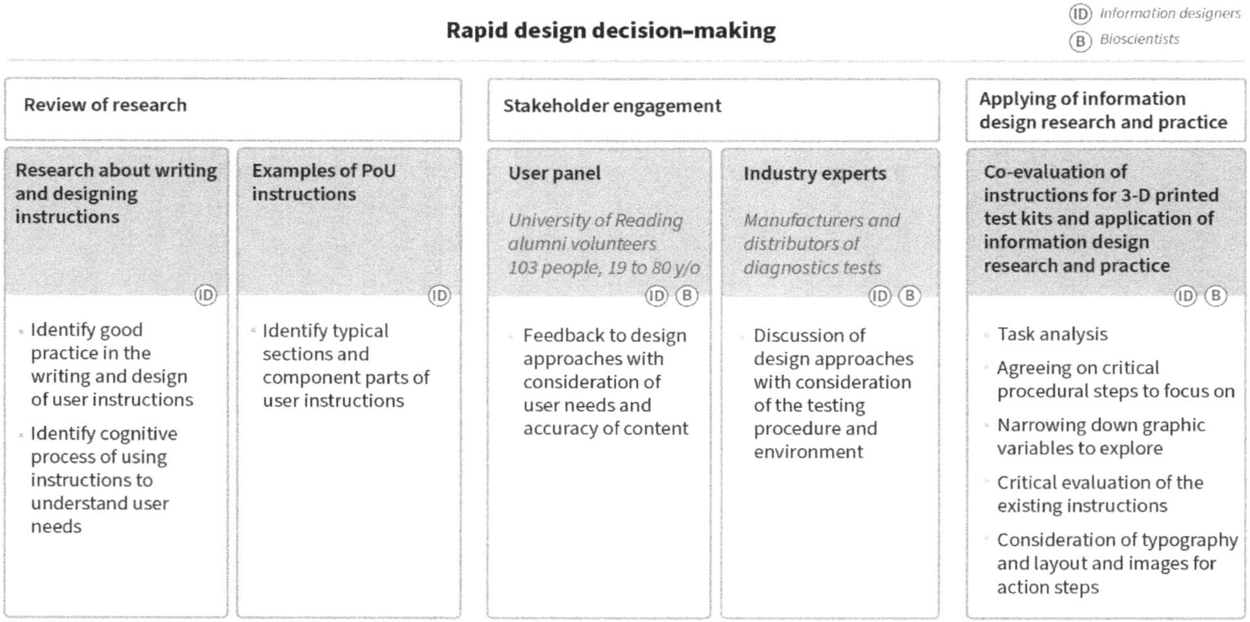

ⒾⒹ *Information designers*
Ⓑ *Bioscientists*

Rapid design decision-making

Review of research		Stakeholder engagement		Applying of information design research and practice
Research about writing and designing instructions ⒾⒹ	**Examples of PoU instructions** ⒾⒹ	**User panel** *University of Reading alumni volunteers 103 people, 19 to 80 y/o* ⒾⒹ Ⓑ	**Industry experts** *Manufacturers and distributors of diagnostics tests* ⒾⒹ Ⓑ	**Co-evaluation of instructions for 3-D printed test kits and application of information design research and practice** ⒾⒹ Ⓑ
▫ Identify good practice in the writing and design of user instructions ▫ Identify cognitive process of using instructions to understand user needs	▫ Identify typical sections and component parts of user instructions	▫ Feedback to design approaches with consideration of user needs and accuracy of content	▫ Discussion of design approaches with consideration of the testing procedure and environment	▫ Task analysis ▫ Agreeing on critical procedural steps to focus on ▫ Narrowing down graphic variables to explore ▫ Critical evaluation of the existing instructions ▫ Consideration of typography and layout and images for action steps

Figure 3.3 Overview of techniques to enable decision-making in the design process (Walker et al., 2022)

The rapid design decision-making has been explained elsewhere (Walker et al., 2022), but exploration of illustration approaches to represent the action steps is summarised below.[4]

Stakeholder engagement: exploring illustration approaches

'Rotate' and 'squeeze' are important and relevant actions in diagnostic LFTs, so as part of our prototype development, we asked our user panel[5] for feedback about different versions showing the use of arrows to denote actions: 'rotate the swab' and 'squeeze the tube'. As part of our iterative design exploration, we invited some members of the panel to explain the meaning of a set of diagrams, and to tell us their preference between alternative approaches. Fourteen people participated (seven women and seven men), who were between 27 and 81 years old. Data were collected using an online questionnaire distributed by email.

- *'Rotate the swab'*. Four versions were designed to indicate 'rotate the swab' in the liquid in the tube (Figure 3.4). The feedback affirmed that all the options conveyed a 'rotation' action overall. However, some participants noted that A and B could be interpreted as 'up and down' or 'back and forth', and that D had an added focus on multiple rotations. The multidimensional arrows C and D were preferred over A and B to represent an action in a three-dimensional space. A further set of diagrams was produced showing the use of a ghosted shape to represent movement, in addition to an arrow (Figure 3.5). Thirteen out of fourteen people preferred a diagram showing the swab in ghosted form. This suggested that using a ghosted shape was effective to explain how to move the swab when no hands were depicted.
- *'Squeeze the tube'*. A further set of diagrams showed four versions of arrows to denote 'squeeze the tube'. There was a clear preference for B, which seemed to be the best for indicating movement (Figure 3.6). It suggests that 'squeeze' is best depicted by vertical gaps in the stem of the arrow rather than changing its shape.

Another factor in the representation of actions is whether it is clearer with no hands, one hand or two hands shown. A set of diagrams

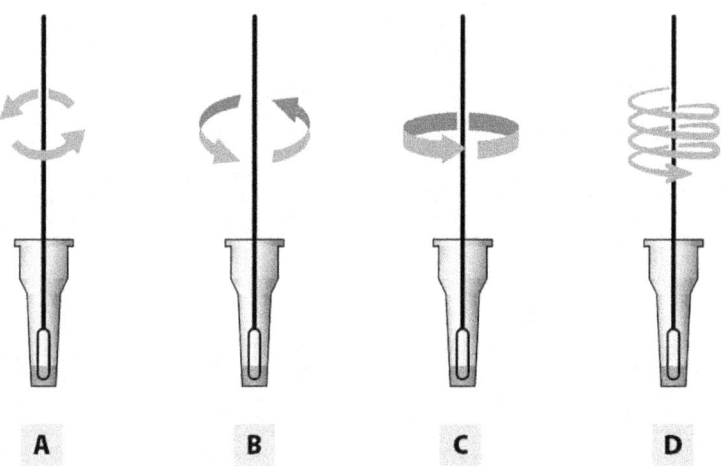

Figure 3.4 Different versions to indicate the action 'rotate the swab'

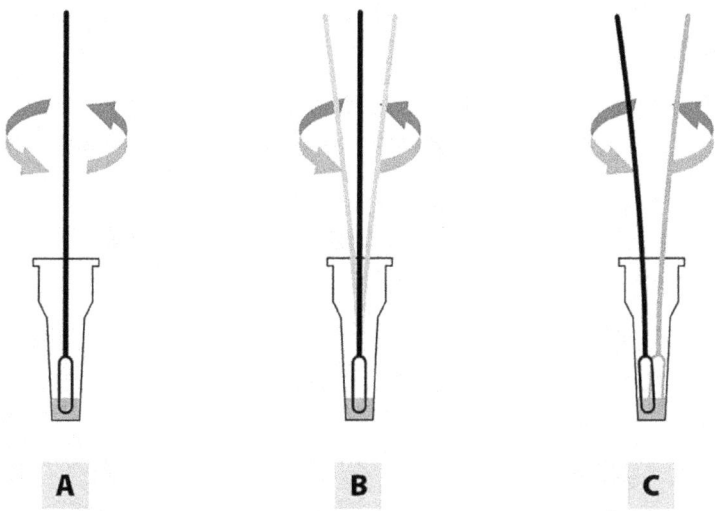

Figure 3.5 Examples B and C show versions of 'rotate the swab' using a ghosted shape

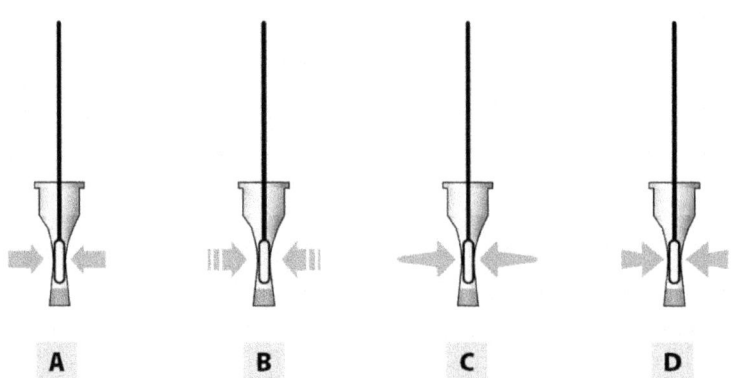

Figure 3.6 Different versions to indicate 'squeeze the tube'

was designed to show the actions 'rotate the swab' and 'squeeze the tube' showing no hands, one hand or two hands (Figure 3.7). There was a clear preference for the use of two hands, suggesting that this is an effective way to embody the action and provide useful information for viewers. This follows existing research on the design of instructional diagrams (Szlichcinski, 1984). As one participant commented: 'The use of hands combined with arrows leaves absolutely no doubt about the intended message'. However, including one or two hands limits the scale at which the tube can be shown, which may make it less easy for users to interpret.

Informal feedback from our user panel and information design good practice were used to make a prototype of new COVID-19

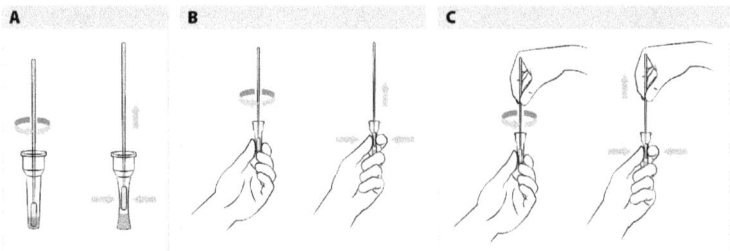

Figure 3.7 Different versions of the actions 'rotate the swab' and 'remove the swab while squeezing the tube' showing the actions with no hand, one or two hands

LFT instructions, shown in Figure 3.8. The action steps are explained through words and pictures, the text is easy to read and colour is used consistently. The sections of the test are clearly identified:

- Set-up information to explain good practice in getting ready to do the test:
  - Items contained in the test kit. This has an inventory function, prompting users to check they have a complete test kit, and helping them to identify each item in advance of using them.
  - Actions to be done before starting the test.
  - An overview of the procedure or a summary of the main goals.
- Instructions for carrying out the test:
  - A step-by-step explanation of actions necessary to complete the test. Includes feedback information so that users can monitor and check their progress.
- Results and what to do next:
  - A clear explanation of what the test results mean and actions to be taken.

The articulation of these principles as shown in Figure 3.8 reflects good information design practice and takes account of the views of our user panel. This panel comprised people with good command of English and with no identified learning needs. For people with specific learning needs, visual impairment or particular language requirements, more work would be needed to ensure that the language used, typography and images took account of this (Hartley, 1994; Leat et al., 2016; NHS England, 2018; Peters et al., 2016; Terras et al., 2021).

Applying the research findings to new circumstances of use and products

We wanted to see how the design of prototype instructions for point-of-use COVID-19 tests could be applied to other kinds of test. We worked with Roche Diagnostics Ltd and the Health Innnovation Agency North West Coast (AHSN) to apply our design approach to

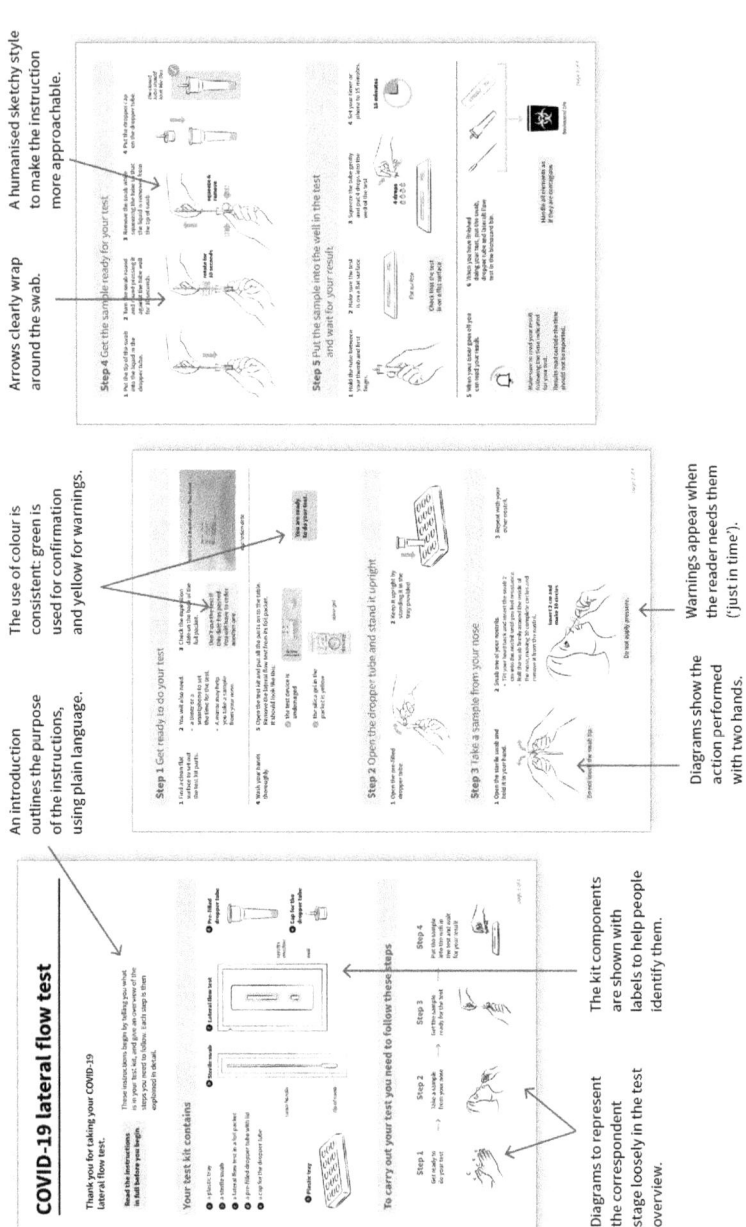

Figure 3.8 Prototype point-of-use instructions for COVID-19 lateral flow tests, developed using evidence from the research project and established knowledge in the design of instructional texts. Annotations refer to use of colour in the prototype (shown here in greyscale).

a set of documents explaining how to use a test for viral flu.[6] Roche and AHSN identified the Standard Operating Procedure (SOP) and Internal Quality Control (IQC) as key texts that needed improvement. The SOP and IQC would be used by health professionals in GP surgeries, outlining the steps they need to follow when administering tests for viral flu so that each patient is treated in a consistent manner, and including instructions for carrying out the test. We agreed to produce user-friendly instructions for a viral flu lateral flow test to form part of a procedural handbook, and a 'quick guide' version that could be positioned, for example, on a wall for easy reference. In applying our approach, we:

- reviewed the manufacturers' regulatory instructions for use to identify the main steps relevant to the Standard Operating Procedure;
- carried out the test to understand the main actions and how to perform them;
- identified the kit components and made drawings in the chosen style;
- drafted wording;
- and set out text and images using the format in our previously-made prototype.

The mode of work was collaborative and iterative: the design team shared successive draft versions with the team at AHSN and Roche Diagnostics. In response, AHSN and Roche team members who were also healthcare workers gave feedback on the structure of the information, the wording and the images. The final version of the SOP is shown in Figure 3.9.[7] The annotations indicate the key things that health professionals carrying out the procedure need to know. These were used as sub-headings, highlighted in orange bands in the document, while the action steps for carrying out the instructions, in this case of lower precedence, are less visually prominent in light blue.

We also produced a 'Quick Guide' version, shown in Figure 3.10, using the same graphic conventions as in the full SOP version, but with edited text and illustrations to include just the key elements. The same approach was applied to the IQC, a procedure that GP surgeries receiving testing kits need to carry out for each box of tests (Figure 3.11).

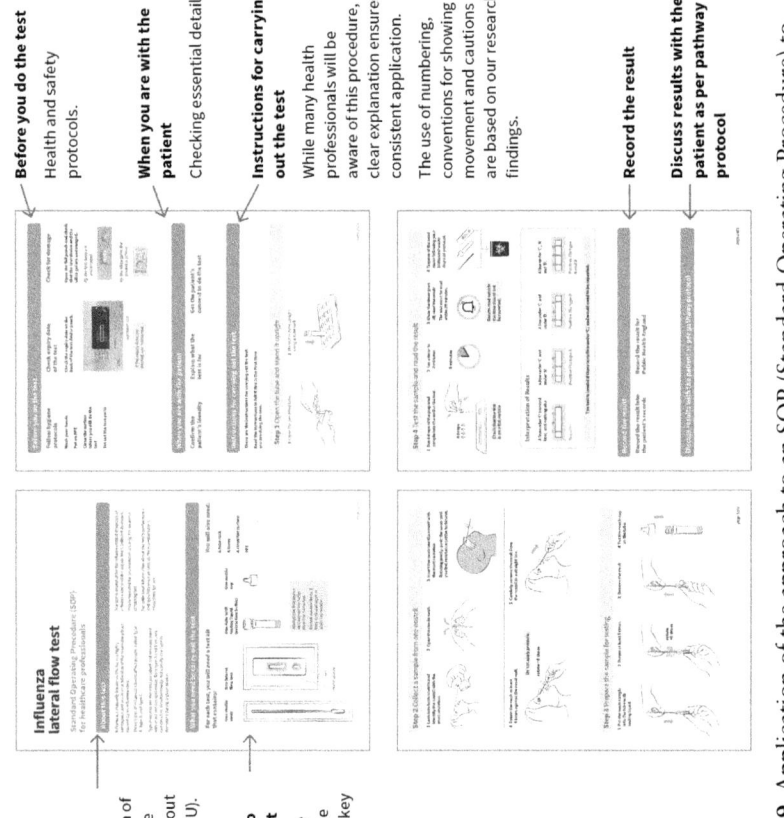

Figure 3.9 Application of the approach to an SOP (Standard Operating Procedure) to operate a lateral flow test for influenza

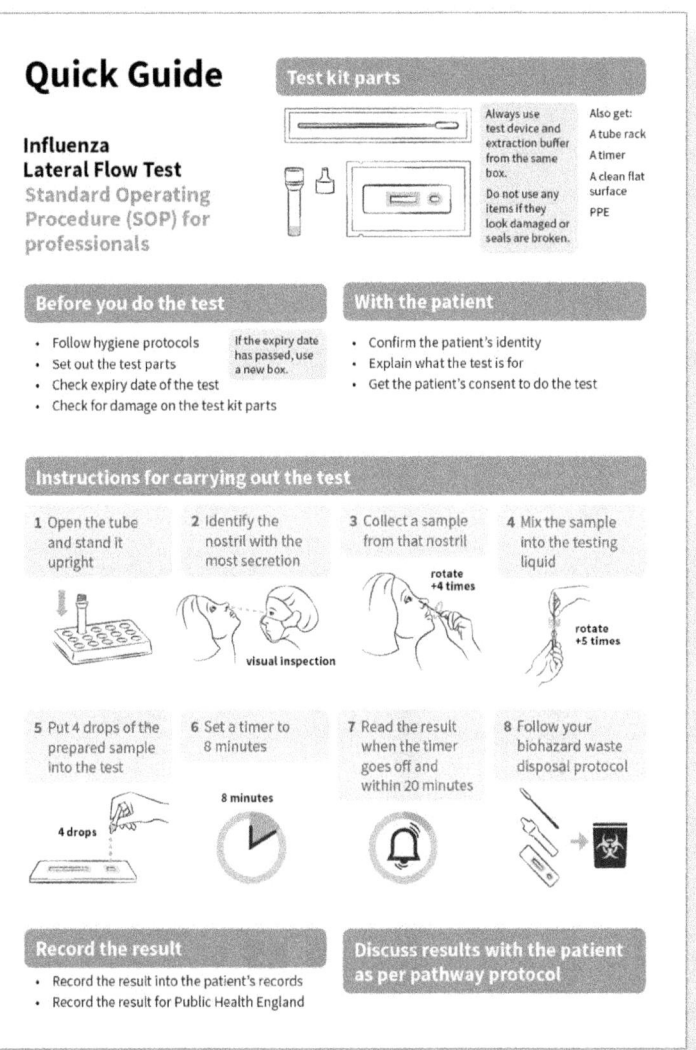

Figure 3.10 SOP Quick Guide, with edited text and illustrations to include the key elements

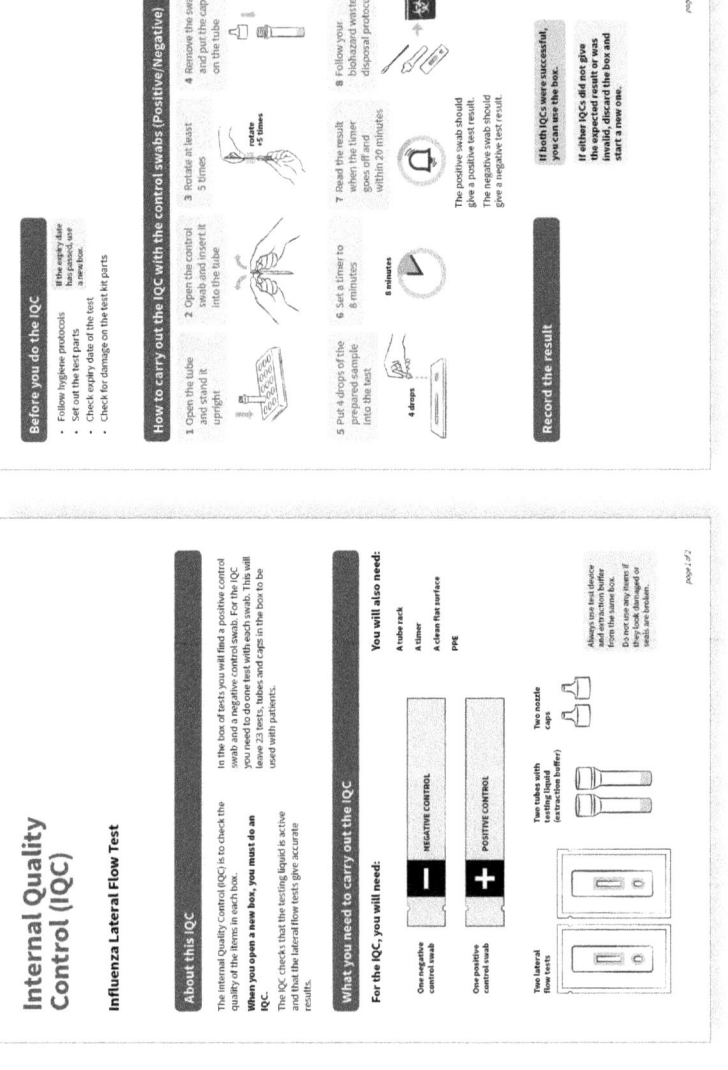

Figure 3.11 Internal Quality Control (IQC), using the same conventions, including horizontal bands to separate the component parts. To distinguish it from the SOP and Quick Guide, a different colour is used for the key steps

The application of our initial prototype demonstrated it could be used effectively as a design template, but while our prototype was most directly applicable to the SOP, variations were required to produce the Quick Guide and the IQC. The underlying principles for organising the information and main components provided a strong starting point; for example, using colour to signal subsets of documents, compressing and simplifying the procedural steps in the Quick Guide, engagement with experts to understand the stages of the protocol and draft simple text and messages accordingly.

A toolkit for making point-of-use instructions

The application of the approach to proposed diagnostic tests for viral flu affirmed our intention to support manufacturers and distributors of tests and service providers to make testing easier and safer. Manufacturers of diagnostic tests are required to follow a regulatory framework for instructions for use. These are detailed and follow British and European principles and general requirements, and tests often include such regulation-required instructions as a pack insert. Previous engagement with manufacturers (by bioscience members of our team) had indicated that traditional Instructions for Use were not seen as easy to use, and there was an appetite for instructions fixed to the principles and guidance of the regulatory framework but made with the needs of users in mind.

We set out to produce an evidence-based practical guide for manufacturers in the form of a toolkit, aimed at diagnostic companies who want to commission point-of-use instructions, and at design professionals who are unfamiliar with the design of procedural instructional text. Similar to instructions for use aimed at the general public, the design guidance needed to be delivered in a way that was quick to search through, easy to understand and simple to apply. We developed an initial draft of the toolkit, to use in semi-structured interviews with regulation implementers and test delivery service providers. The aim was to gauge industry views about the focus and relevance of our approach.

Five professionals in point-of-care diagnostics were contacted through professional networks. All were working in the UK, developing and/or providing service delivery of different types of tests, including lateral flow tests. Semi-structured interviews were conducted online to understand whether they and their companies recognised the importance of point-of-use instructions, and to explore what guidance they would find helpful.[8] The interview was structured in two stages:

- Initial questions aimed to establish their views about the role of user instructions (*'How much attention does your organisation/you pay to instructions for diagnostic tests* [for home use]*?'*, *'Do you review the instructions that come with the test* [i.e., the manufacturers' instructions for use] *before distribution? Why?' 'Can you explain what you're looking for?' 'What do you do if the instructions look unacceptable?'*).
- Then, interviewees were shown sample pages of the draft toolkit, and asked about the perceived usefulness of such an approach (*'We are producing a set of guidelines – a toolkit – to explain how to produce Point of Use instructions. This is an example. How would something like this work for you? What is missing? What do you like about this and why?'*)

Due to the small number of interviews, the responses were transcribed and recurrent views were summarised. It is not assumed that these views represent all manufacturers and service providers. However, the contributions of interviewees inform our understanding of competing requirements that affect the way in which crucial user information is communicated to non-expert audiences that operate the tests.

Suitability of IFUs for lay users – When discussing the suitability of IFUs for lay users, there was widespread recognition of the difference in purpose and audience between IFUs and point-of-use instructions, and that IFUs are not designed to be first and foremost easy to use. There was general understanding that instructions for expert and non-expert users have different requirements, and that information that would satisfy the regulator would not necessarily satisfy the non-expert final user. One interviewee commented: 'There are plenty of regulatory requirements which I don't think add value to the end user, but are required from a legal standpoint, definitely.'

Initial reactions to toolkit approach – When shown draft sample pages from the toolkit, interviewees' comments suggested that the content was relevant and could be used by members of the industry looking to produce user-friendly instructions: 'it provides a really good framework from which to start'; 'it's really valuable work' and 'I am absolutely certain that what you've done is useful'. The sample pages included recommendations about plain language, short text and clear diagrams, which the interviewees agreed with and highlighted as important points to get across. Perhaps unsurprisingly, interviewees supported the use of illustrations to assist with explanation and remarked that long text is likely to dissuade readers from engaging. They pointed out that clear diagrams are important to make the instructions inclusive; for example, for people with different reading and cognitive abilities, and for speakers of English as a second language.

Important aspects to include – When asked for further aspects to cover in the toolkit, two interviewees pointed out that point-of-use instructions should communicate the implications of possible errors for the final user. There was a sense that, in addition to showing the correct actions, good instructions should be clear about key actions, the implications of not doing them and include warnings and troubleshooting. Two participants commented: 'You're not telling people just what to do, you're trying to avoid key errors as well', and 'sometimes, the people who design [these tests] give very little information about the impact of not doing something'.

The resulting feedback has been incorporated into a toolkit comprising three main sections, which provide guidance on engaging with intended users, treating content and structure and using illustrations and text in point-of-use instructions (Figure 3.12). The purpose of the toolkit is to:

- encourage test manufacturers and suppliers to consider point-of-use when creating instructional documentation for their tests;
- support manufacturers and distributors of tests in the preparation of point-of-use instructions to suit specific audiences and circumstances of use;
- and implement user-centred design research and practice in producing instructional documentation for users.

The recommendations are supplemented by references to existing research, examples of how the guidance has been applied to non-COVID instructions and examples of good practice in procedural instructions (Walker, Bravo and Edwards, 2022).

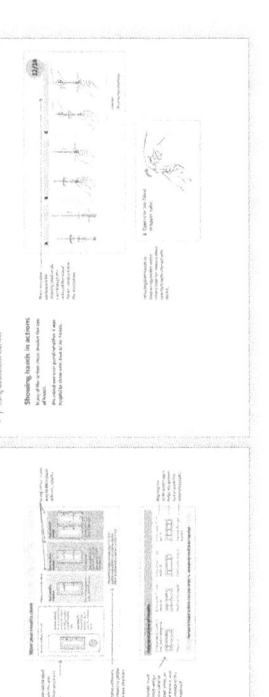

Figure 3.12 Pages of the toolkit 'User-friendly point-of-use instructions for home use diagnostic tests: guidance and tools'. Each page in the toolkit summarises key issues and provides captioned or annotated illustrations to explain the key points

Research-informed guidelines such as the toolkit can raise the profile of point-of-use instructions and support the creation of user-friendly instructions. However, guidelines are, by nature, non-prescriptive and hence open to interpretation.[9] Even if design guidelines are followed to create point-of-use instructions, some form of testing with end users is required to assess whether the resulting document meets the users' needs. While end users have been involved throughout our project, we have not yet taken full account of specific user requirements, including the needs of final users of instructions for whom English is not a first language, older people and people who are partially sighted. Engagement with such groups would most likely result in different prototype solutions, perhaps with text in two languages and captioned images; or with adjusted typography. The underlying principles in the toolkit would be relevant in helping the design decision-making in relation to such user groups.

Concluding remarks

Our investigation into the design of procedural instructions for diagnostic tests has identified the critical importance of these instructions, noted some barriers and complexities and delivered a framework for future community test products. Our work has not only affirmed the need for and value of instructions at point-of-use, but also provides insight into why these are especially important for community testing.

When our project started, COVID-19 home testing was becoming part of everyday life, and instructions for carrying out tests were being produced by professionals, by lay people and in a number of formats. While such instructions enabled people to carry out tests effectively at point-of-use, research into the effectiveness of COVID-19 rapid tests drew attention to parts of the test that were especially vulnerable to procedural errors, and that could result in invalid results. Our research investigated how to represent some of the actions – such as rotate a swab and squeeze out a specified number of drops – that people found difficult in the context of carrying out an LFT at home. The resulting prototype for instructions drew on this research and applied established information design good practice.

Our research-informed guidance for producing point-of-use instructions – in the form of a toolkit – aims to help diagnostic test manufacturers and service providers produce user-friendly instructions. The key messages in the toolkit are: work with users and get their feedback about draft versions; keep key messages straightforward and clear; and use images to help explain procedures. This toolkit exemplifies what is 'good design' for user-friendly procedural instructions.

The time is right for such guidance, not least because of a likely increase in the use of home- or community-use diagnostic testing kits going forward. For some respiratory infections, such as COVID-19 or influenza, antiviral drugs can significantly reduce disease severity, and home treatment is possible as these are administered orally. Crucially, treatment is only effective if the correct drug is administered soon after symptoms start. Lateral flow tests from saliva or swabs have therefore great potential to target antiviral drugs specifically to vulnerable patients.

The project did not focus on ways to change regulation on IFUs. Our approach was to explore ways to meet the needs of patients by producing documents targeted at specific audiences. For example, in applying our approach to the SOP for viral flu, the decision was made early on not to interfere with the traditional SOP (containing regulatory information) and, instead, produce visually informative documents that could be used at point-of-use, and inserted into the larger documentation for reference. However, an increase in point-of-care testing will need to go hand-in-hand with instructions made with final users in mind. Our conversations with members of the industry suggest that clashing requirements of regulation and final users are acknowledged, but time constraints in manufacturing and approval processes mean that meeting the regulations is prioritised over clear patient- or user-facing communication. Collaborative work between graphic communication designers and designers of medical devices may be a way forward to align products to the needs of regulators and patients.

Notes

1 The widespread community use significantly pre-dated full publication of extensive field validation and especially full usability studies exploring the user experience (Dinnes et al., 2021), and only much later was it possible to fully review multiple studies.
2 See our 'research briefings' at https://research.reading.ac.uk/design-research-for-testing-diagnostics/three-research-briefings-to-inform-the-design-of-instructions-for-covid-tests/
3 Information design has an established academic track record (as projected by Stiff, 2005; and see also Black et al., 2017).
4 See https://research.reading.ac.uk/design-research-for-testing-diagnostics/ for detail about these studies.
5 We recruited a user panel under terms of reference that complied with the research ethics requirements of the funded research. A group of University of Reading alumni volunteers agreed to be part of a user panel. The panel comprised 102 people (68 women and 34 men) between 19 and 80 years old. This panel agreed to be part of an iterative design review process providing feedback or comments. For each iteration, panel members were asked to answer an online questionnaire, a COVID-necessary format. See Walker et al. (2022).
6 A team from Roche Diagnostics collaborated in the original research project, offering insights from the manufacturer/distributor perspective. The team from Roche Diagnostics proposed and initiated the application of the prototype instructions to tests for viral flu.
7 The design process was collaborative, involving designers and industry colleagues. As noted by Shirley Shinkfield, from the Health Innovation Agency North West Coast: 'Initial discussions took place to outline the project requirements, and from that point the Innovation Agency were kept updated and involved via emails and meetings as the design process evolved, ensuring the final product was fit for purpose and importantly user friendly for the intended audience (multi-disciplinary healthcare staff)'.
8 This work was funded by the University of Reading's Rapid Response Policy Engagement funding from Research England.
9 As noted by Pat Wright (2003: 9): 'Simple design guidelines will never be adequate for patient information because achieving success often means resolving design conflicts. Successful compromises need to be based on a broad and detailed knowledge of design options and their consequences for readers.' See also Raynor and Dickinson (2009).

References

Atchison, C., Pristerà, P., Cooper, E., et al. (2020), Usability and acceptability of home-based self-testing for SARS-CoV-2 antibodies for population surveillance. *Clinical Infectious Diseases*, 72(9). https://doi.org/10.1093/cid/ciaa1178

Black, A., Lund, O. and Walker, S., eds (2017), *Information Design: Research and Practice*. Abingdon: Routledge.

BMJ. (2021), Performance of the Innova SARS-CoV-2 antigen rapid lateral flow test in the Liverpool asymptomatic testing pilot: Population based cohort study. *British Medical Journal*, 374, n1637. https://doi.org/10.1136/bmj.n1637

Cherne, N., Moses, R., Piperato, S. M., et al. (2020), How medical device instructions for use engage users. *Biomedical Instrumentation and Technology*, 54(4), 258–268. https://doi.org/10.2345/0899-8205-54.4.258

Dickinson, D. and Gallina, S. (2017), 'Information Design in Medicine Package Leaflets' in A. Black, O. Lund and S. Walker (eds), *Information Design: Research and Practice*. London: Routledge, pp. 685–700.

Dinnes, J., Deeks, J. J., Berhane, S., et al. (2021), Rapid, point-of-care antigen tests for diagnosis of SARS-CoV-2 infection. *Cochrane Database of Systematic Reviews*, 3, CD013705. doi: 10.1002/14651858.CD013705.pub2

gov.uk. (2021), Press release. Available at: www.gov.uk/government/news/9-in-10-pharmacies-now-offering-free-rapid-coronavirus-covid-19-tests

Hartley, J. (1994), Designing instructional text for older readers: A literature review. *British Journal of Educational Technology*, 25(3), 172–188.

IEEE, IEC and ISO. (2019). Preparation of information for use (instructions for use) of products: Principles and general requirements. IEC/IEEE 82079-1 (ISO standard).

Kierkegaard, P., McLister, A. and Buckle, P. (2021), Rapid point-of-care testing for COVID-19: Quality of supportive information for lateral flow serology assays. *BMJ Open*, 11(3), e047163. https://doi.org/10.1136/bmjopen-2020-047163

Leat, S. J., Krishnamoorthy, A., Carbonara, A., et al. (2016), Improving the legibility of prescription medication labels for older adults and adults with visual impairment. *Canadian Pharmacists Journal*, 149(3), 174–184. https://doi.org/10.1177/1715163516641432

Needs, S. H., Bull, S. P., Bravo, J., et al. (2020), Remote videolink observation of model home sampling and home testing devices to simplify usability studies for point-of-care diagnostics. *Wellcome Open Research*, 5, 174. https://doi.org/10.12688/wellcomeopenres.16105.1

NHS England. (2018), Guide to making information accessible for people with a learning disability. Available at: www.england.nhs.uk/publication/guide-to-making-information-accessible-for-people-with-a-learning-disability/

Peters, P., Smith, A., Funk, Y., et al. (2016). Language, terminology and the readability of online cancer information. *Medical Humanities*, 42(1), 36–41. https://doi.org/10.1136/medhum-2015-010766

Raynor, David K. and Dickinson, David (2009), Key principles to guide development of consumer medicine information: Content analysis of information design texts. *The Annals of Pharmacotherapy*, 43, 700–709.

St John, A. and Price, C. P. (2014), Existing and emerging technologies for point-of-care testing. *Clinical Biochemist Reviews*, 35(3), 155–167.

Stiff, P. (2005), Some documents for a history of information design. *Information Design Journal*, 13(2), 216–228.

Szlichcinski, C. (1984), 'Factors Affecting the Comprehension of Pictographic Instructions' in R. Easterby and H. Zwaga (eds), *Information Design* . Chichester: John Wiley and Sons, pp. 449–466.

Terras, M. M., Jarrett, D. and McGregor, S. A. (2021), The importance of accessible information in promoting the inclusion of people with an intellectual disability. *Disabilities*, 1(3), 132–150. https://doi.org/10.3390/disabilities1030011

Tong, V., Raynor, D. K. and Aslani, P. (2014), Design and comprehensibility of over-the-counter product labels and leaflets: A narrative review. *International Journal of Clinical Pharmacy*, 36(5), 865–872. https://doi.org/10.1007/s11096-014-9975-0

Walker, S. (2017), 'The Contribution of Typography and Information Design to Health Communications' in E. Tsekleves and R. Cooper (eds), *Design for Health*. New York: Routledge, pp. 92–109.

Walker, S. (2019), Effective antimicrobial resistance communication: The role of information design. *Palgrave Communications*, 5(1). https://doi.org/10.1057/s41599-019-0231-z

Walker, S., Bravo, J., Edwards, A., et al. (2022), *User-friendly point-of-use instructions for home use diagnostic tests*. Other. University of Reading doi: https://doi.org/10.17864/1947.000419

Waller, R. and VandenBerg, S. (2017), A one-day transformation project for overdose emergency kits. *Information Design Journal*, 23(3), 319–333. https://doi.org/10.1075/idj.23.3.05wal

Wright, P. (2003), Criteria and ingredients for successful patient information. *Journal of Audiovisual Media in Medicine*, 26(1), 6–10

4

Home and neighbourhood: Pandemic geographies of dwelling and belonging

Alison Blunt, Kathy Burrell, Georgina Endfield, Miri Lawrence, Eithne Nightingale, Alastair Owens, Jacqueline Waldock and Annabelle Wilkins

The home has been at the forefront of political and public health responses to, and people's lives during, the COVID-19 pandemic. National directives in many countries to 'stay home', alongside border closures and other restrictions, limited local and transnational mobility to an unprecedented extent (Blunt and Dowling, 2022; Fitzgerald, 2020). In the UK there were three periods of nationwide lockdown in 2020 (March–May, November–December) and 2021 (January–March) when the majority of the population faced significant limitations on leaving their places of residence (see Institute for Government, 2022, for full details of lockdowns and other forms of restriction across the UK and its devolved nations). People experienced the impact of the universal directive to 'stay home' in very different ways, as explored by a growing body of research on home and everyday life during the pandemic that spans critiques of the limited and exclusionary assumptions about home, household and family (Grewal et al., 2020; Sophie Lewis, 2020); home-working and home-schooling (Aznar et al., 2021; Dimopoulos et al., 2021; Islam, 2022); the rise of domestic violence and abuse (Piquero et al., 2021; Women's Aid, 2020); the impact of the pandemic on migrant domestic workers (Pandey et al., 2021; Rao et al., 2021); digital connectivity in the home (Maalsen and Dowling, 2020); the effects of housing precarity and design on mental health, wellbeing and domestic life (Alonso and Jacoby, 2023; Bower et al., 2023; Erfani and Bahrami, 2023; Preece et al., 2023; Waldron, 2023); and religious faith and practice at home during the pandemic (Bryson et al., 2020; Lawrence et al., 2022).

Across this wide-ranging and growing field of research on home and COVID-19, new forms of connection and disconnection with people and places beyond the household and the domestic dwelling have emerged as important themes. Drawing on research conducted as part of the AHRC-funded Stay Home Stories project (www.stayhomestories.co.uk), and informed by wider research on what Blunt and Sheringham (2019) term 'home-city geographies', this chapter explores pandemic geographies of dwelling and belonging on domestic and neighbourhood scales for UK residents in London and Liverpool. In so doing, it extends broader debates about urban homes as sites of dis/connection with the wider neighbourhood (Sheringham et al., 2023) and interactions with neighbours and neighbourhoods during the COVID-19 pandemic (Mehta, 2020; Ottoni et al., 2022; Preece et al., 2023). In this chapter we address three key questions: how were people's 'stay home' lives shaped by interactions with their neighbours and neighbourhoods? How did such interactions shape people's pandemic experiences of dwelling and belonging on domestic and neighbourhood scales? What insights can we take forward to shape fairer home-city futures? Throughout, we argue that the home – porous and bounded, expansive and confined – is a site of pandemic dis/connection with the wider neighbourhood. Homes and neighbourhoods were formative in shaping people's lived experiences of COVID-19 and visions for the future of both should be a central part of local and national pandemic recovery agendas. We begin by situating our research within wider debates about urban homes and neighbourhoods.

Urban homes and neighbourhoods

Through their analysis of a series of pre-pandemic 'home-city biographies' with residents in Hackney, east London, Sheringham et al. (2023) argue that home is a site of connection and disconnection with the wider urban neighbourhood and city. By taking a 'home-city geographies' approach, which explores the connections between urban domesticities (home in the city) and domestic urbanism (the city as home), they draw attention 'to the importance of people's domestic lives in their sense of belonging (or not belonging) to the neighbourhood and wider city', highlighting 'the role of urban encounters – with immediate neighbours and in the wider neighbourhood – in people's experiences of home, which may involve a feeling of *isolation* from, or of being *part* of, something larger' (Sheringham et al., 2023: 733; see also Blunt and Sheringham, 2019; Burrell, 2014). By foregrounding the intertwined geographies of home, neighbourhood and the wider city, Sheringham et al. (2023) develop broader debates about urban conviviality, the contested domestication of urban space and neighbourly and neighbourhood interactions. In contrast to research that explores living together in the city largely, and often exclusively, in relation to 'lives lived in urban public space' (2023: 722), Sheringham et al. argue that it is

> only by taking seriously the practices, experiences and imaginings of home as a site of connection and/or disconnection with neighbours, neighbourhoods, and the wider city that … urban scholars can gain a full picture of what it means to live together in the city, and to understand some of the inequalities, exclusions and prejudices that shape urban lives. (Sheringham et al., 2023: 719)

Sheringham et al. further stress the temporal dynamics of dis/connections between home and the urban neighbourhood, whereby 'the experiences and narratives of home *in* the city, and the city *as* home, ebb and flow over time' (2023: 733), bound up with personal, familial and household changes over the life course, alongside wider processes of urban change (Blunt et al., 2020). From March 2020, 'stay home' directives and other restrictions in response to the COVID-19 pandemic in the UK and many other countries marked a significant and unprecedented disjuncture in the interplay of personal and urban temporalities. Three national lockdowns in 2020 and 2021 – and other periods of restriction, including in the north east and north west of England from August to October 2020 and via tiered systems across the UK – not only limited contact with people beyond the household – or, from June 2020, beyond a household 'bubble' for people living alone or single parents – but also limited the amount of time that most people, except key workers, could spend outside their homes (Institute for Government, 2022). Alongside travel restrictions within and beyond the UK, this meant that people spent a far greater amount of time within their local neighbourhoods.

Writing at an early point in the pandemic, Vikas Mehta explored what he termed 'the new proxemics', whereby people – particularly those living in mid-to low-density places – were 'experiencing their neighbourhoods differently' (2020: 669). While recognising stark social disparities, Mehta wrote that 'social distancing has delivered, in many neighbourhoods, a new and *sociable* space' (2020: 669), reflecting a wider desire under tight restrictions for 'the publicness of the everyday – socializing, conversations and other interactions with our neighbours and others' (Mehta, 2020: 670). Alongside quantitative research on the spatial and social disparities in the decline of activities at the neighbourhood scale during the pandemic and its impact on rates of infection (Trasberg and Cheshire, 2023), other research has explored people's lived experiences of neighbourhoods and their relationships with their neighbours. Ottoni et al. (2022), for example, analyse interviews conducted with older residents in Vancouver from March to June 2020 to explore the importance of 'social connectedness', both with neighbours in their apartment buildings and in their wider neighbourhood. Recognising the impact of 'unneighbourliness' on the 'unmaking of home' (Baxter and Brickell, 2014; Cheshire et al., 2021), Preece et al. (2023: 1658) explain that 'close proximity to others demonstrates how the practices of one neighbour can impede the home-making of another', particularly through noise (also see Alonso and Jacoby, 2023). Within the neighbourhood, many researchers have stressed the importance of access to domestic and public green spaces during the pandemic for mental and physical health and wellbeing, particularly for people living in overcrowded and sub-standard housing (Burnett et al., 2021; Dobson, 2021; Erfani and Bahrami, 2023; Foster, 2020; and Mell and Whitten, 2021), while recognising the unevenness of access to them, due in part to park closures at the start of the first national lockdown (Blunt et al., 2022; Foster, 2020). This chapter contributes to this wider research through its focus on both home and neighbourhood, and the encounters with neighbours that played a significant part in deepening or limiting experiences of the neighbourhood as home during the height of the pandemic. By bringing pre-pandemic work on home-city dis/connections into dialogue with research on neighbourhoods and neighbourly interactions during the pandemic, we seek to 'know the pandemic' by understanding people's 'stay home' lives and their ideas about home on domestic, neighbourhood and urban scales. To do so, we draw on interviews conducted in London and Liverpool as part of the Stay Home Stories project.

Stay Home Stories

Stay Home Stories is a collaborative research project based at the Centre for Studies of Home, a partnership between Queen Mary University of London and Museum of the Home, and conducted with the University of Liverpool, the Royal Geographical Society (with the Institute of British Geographers) and National Museums Liverpool. The research project had three main aims: first, to document and analyse the ways in which home has been mobilised, experienced and imagined during and after three UK national lockdowns; to explore and extend creative and curatorial work that documents diverse experiences and imaginings of home; and to understand how practices, spaces and meanings of home have changed during and after lockdown, particularly for adults from different ethnic, migration and faith backgrounds and for children and young people. The research has involved more than 100 online interviews with adults living in London and Liverpool – two cities with particularly high rates of COVID-19 at different times in the pandemic (see Blunt et al., 2022; Burrell et al., 2021) – as well as the analysis of more than 400 maps of home during the pandemic drawn by children and young people aged 7 to 16 throughout the UK. Project outputs – all available at www.stayhomestories.co.uk – include reports on home and COVID-19 in London and Liverpool (Blunt et al., 2022; Burrell et al., 2021); a report on the impact of the pandemic on artists (Nightingale et al., 2022); a resource guide for people of faith (Lawrence et al., 2022); a series of short films and podcasts; teaching resources; and blog posts. We include two maps from our research in this chapter, and more can be seen in an online gallery (www.rgs.org/schools/projects-and-partnerships/stay-home-rethinking-the-domestic-during-the-covid-19-pandemic/mapping-home) hosted by the Royal Geographical Society (with the Institute of British Geographers).

Aged between 18 and 73, our interviewees came from a wide range of ethnic, migration and faith backgrounds, and worked in a variety of sectors. Some worked from home during the pandemic or were on a temporary absence from work under the furlough scheme, while others, including key workers, continued to work beyond the home. Some participants have lived in London or Liverpool for all or most of their lives, while others have moved there more recently. Participants lived in a variety of housing types (terraced, semi-detached and detached houses; flats; and student accommodation), tenures (social housing, rented and privately owned accommodation) and households (alone, with family members, or in shared accommodation with friends or flat-mates). Many of our participants were recruited and interviewed by community researchers working on the project in Liverpool and east London, as well as by other members of the project team. Reflecting the wider research aims, interview questions spanned a range of topics including: changes to people's households and domestic practices during COVID-19; relationships with family and friends; experiences of being and feeling at home in the local neighbourhood; migrant homes in pandemic times; and the impacts of coronavirus restrictions on religious belief and practice.

Pandemic homes and neighbourhoods

Local neighbourhoods came to be increasingly significant for many of our interviewees during the pandemic, particularly during periods of lockdown.[1] Alexandra describes, for example, her experience of living in Liverpool shrinking to her neighbourhood when, after a few bike rides to the city centre early in the first lockdown, she remained closer to home:

> [T]he city has felt much smaller, for sure ... my world has felt really small ... there is a sense of living in a village... I don't live in a city at the moment. I haven't lived in the city for a while. It's quite a small village that I live in.

Even as her everyday life in the city became more localised, Alexandra describes her growing identification of Liverpool as home during the pandemic, mainly because she chose to remain there rather than return to Athens to work remotely:

> I think it was during the pandemic that I realised Liverpool is home... I know quite a few people that live in the UK mainly and they went back to Athens during the pandemic. And because being able to work from anywhere, just gives you the option. And I really wanted to go last summer and spend a lot of time there. But ... it makes me realise that it's here, like that's where I am. That's where home is and I'm not here because of work ... I choose to be here. So, I think that's the main thing that changed during the pandemic, like this question of where home is was resolved ... by making this choice of where to be, where you have the option to be. To be isolated, to be stuck at the place. Where do you choose to be stuck?

For Alexandra, this wider sense of Liverpool as home was rooted in her neighbourhood:

> [T]his area of Liverpool, from Sefton Park to Toxteth is – that's where home is... [T]hat has been clear to me when I say Liverpool is home, which part of Liverpool I mean. And the country? I can't say that like England is home or the UK. So, it's very localised. It's Liverpool (see also Blunt and Bonnerjee (2013) and Bonnerjee (2012) on diasporic attachments to cities and neighbourhoods as home).

Many people described how their relationships with local places and communities became stronger during the COVID-19 pandemic. Cuong, for example, moved to Woolwich in London shortly before lockdown and began to view his neighbourhood as a place to 'live a bit more' rather than 'a place to store clothes and sleep'. Julie valued her Tower Hamlets neighbourhood in London for its diversity and inclusivity: 'everybody feels when they're here they belong here, and that's great because it's very inclusive of everybody and that's the best thing about it.... I think it's one of the few places in the world where people always feel at home ... wherever they're from.' She also appreciated its amenities and connections to other places in the city:

> Although I'm in the heart of the city or the heart of London, I'm also next to quite rural spaces like the City Farm, Allen Gardens and other sort[s] of local parks. I have really good facilities for transport

near me so it's easy to get to, also I've got local high streets near me all in walking distance... So it's very connected, and I think this is one of the reasons why lots of people come to live here ... because it's one of the most really connected places.

Farah, who had moved to Walthamstow in London before the pandemic, felt more rooted in her neighbourhood and local community:

> I definitely grew to like my neighbourhood much, much more, because ... when I moved to this neighbourhood I thought ... I don't know anything about it... But during the pandemic I realised like I made it home here and I really want to stay here, because I really liked the general community, and liked the approach to community.

But while many people felt more strongly rooted in their neighbourhoods and local communities during the pandemic, others felt increasingly disconnected. Miriam, for example, felt that both her house and Liverpool were home, alongside where her parents and other family members live in Spain, but missed a sense of community in her neighbourhood and felt lonely and isolated during the pandemic:

> It's a really nice area with nice views and that, but there is no sense of community at all. Because we have just some ... big blocks, lots of hotels and office spaces. So there is not local shops that are close. There is not a local market, there is not a local park. There is not a space for neighbours to be together really... I would prefer to live in an area with a greater sense of community, definitely. I think it's more rewarding. It makes you feel more integrated in society really. I felt really, really lonely during lockdown. I felt really lonely. And if I had had more friends or closer neighbours, that wouldn't have been ... so bad for me... I felt if something happened to me, nobody would realise or nobody would come. I mean my family is in Spain so they couldn't fly. I couldn't go there... It's funny how the house was suddenly like too small. I'm always ok there and suddenly the house was too small. And I was lonely, and I'm always alone and I love it.

While Miriam had previously enjoyed living alone, her lack of local friends, neighbours and wider sense of community made her feel isolated and vulnerable during pandemic restrictions. She experienced loneliness not only on a domestic scale but also in relation to her wider neighbourhood. Her experiences are revealing of the limitations of public health 'stay home' directives, which appear predicated on particular assumptions about domestic relations and urban sociality that are not achievable for everyone. As Sheringham et al. observe, 'While the literature on urban conviviality focuses on living together in urban public space, much of the literature on loneliness focuses on people living alone and emphasizes *household* rather than *home*', obscuring 'a broader understanding of the multiple material and social factors that contribute to the experience of feeling at home or not at home', including those beyond the domestic dwelling from neighbourhood to transnational scales (Sheringham et al., 2023: 723). Alongside her loneliness within her home and neighbourhood, Miriam, like many other participants with family and friends in other countries, also found international travel restrictions very difficult:

> [I]t was disturbing, the idea of not being able to fly if needed from one home to the other one. Because I mean Liverpool is my home, but I know I can take a flight whenever I need it and be here [in Spain] in a couple of hours. And the idea of not being able to do it was really disturbing (also see Burrell et al., 2021).

Other participants reflected on the relationships between their homes and neighbourhoods in different ways. Salma, for example, described her sense of home as wherever she was with her fiancé, dog and cat, but found that during periods of lockdown and other restrictions,

> I had a difficult relationship with home because this is home, but ... I felt trapped a lot of the time ... home didn't feel like a comfortable space anymore ... home felt forced and I felt like I was trapped a lot of the time, and I felt like I couldn't go out ... everything felt really restrictive, even though ... you could go on a walk. So it wasn't like I was completely trapped in a house, but I felt trapped in my little place... I did feel like I was at home, but I didn't feel like it was comforting.

Salma's experiences of home – vividly conveyed through her reiteration of feeling 'trapped' – were closely bound up with the limitations of her Liverpool neighbourhood as a place to live during the pandemic. Before the pandemic, Salma and her fiancé had moved to a neighbourhood with good transport connections because travelling had been an important part of their work:

> Although the neighbourhood is not a bad neighbourhood in particular, there are definitely better neighbourhoods I think that we could have selected based on being at home more. So when we bought this house, we picked it based on our career trajectories at that point ... it did what it needed to do, but then when we did go into lockdown ... I remember saying to my fiancé I wish we had a bigger garden or I wish we had more space or I wish we lived ... closer to a shop. Because where we live, we have to drive to a shop, there is nowhere, I think there's a corner shop about a mile and a half away, but literally there isn't anything really ... it's quite enclosed. There are just houses here and there's a motorway just sort of down the road-ish.

Salma and many other participants talked about the importance of gardens, parks and other outdoor spaces to sustain them during lockdowns and other restrictions. While access to private and shared gardens helped people cope with the restrictions of lockdown on a domestic scale, access to local parks and other outside spaces were crucial in helping people to feel more at home in their wider neighbourhood (also see Vertovec (2015), on urban 'rooms without walls', including parks, in New York, Singapore and Johannesburg). Local parks and other outside spaces took on an enhanced significance in many people's lives, not least because they offered, as one participant put it, a break from 'being confined inside' and 'just something different than being [inside] ... the same four walls again'. In research conducted before the pandemic, Sheringham et al. (2023) describe the importance of views from windows, doors and balconies in understanding residents' connections between their home and urban neighbourhood. Views of – as well as access to – green space and water were particularly important during lockdown restrictions.

For Miriam, who felt lonely and isolated in her home and neighbourhood, having a terrace (on a balcony) was a crucial way of feeling connected to nature and the outdoors during lockdown:

> I think my outdoor space, my terrace, is definitely more valued than ever. No, no, it's always been an important part of the house and

I didn't realise. Because I have really big glass windows. So even if I'm working all day, because I can have a look at the outside world, it's also really relaxing because I have water, there's this lake, I have birds and stuff. I can see the sunset. So it feels like I am outside. So sometimes I will spend three or four days at home without realising that I haven't been out.

Living near Liverpool's waterfront was important for Luis who moved to the city from Malta:

We're Mediterraneans and we come from an island, and we're used to seeing and living by the water. And that is, at least to me, comforting ... from my living room, I can see water and I can see the docks, and I can see the river, and I can see the tide. And also, if I walk, if I get out of the house, I'm immediately by the water, although it's a different type of water than, you know, Mediterranean waters, but it's still satisfying in a way and then we go for walks along the waterfront.

The importance of green spaces beyond the home was also a prominent theme in the maps drawn by children and young people. Niccolo's map of home in London during the pandemic (Figure 4.1), for example, focuses predominantly on places beyond the home – including shops, school and a church – and places particular emphasis on parks, the River Thames, trees and wildlife. His house is positioned centrally amidst these different features of the local neighbourhood, but the map focuses more on what is beyond the house than what is inside, highlighting the importance of urban green-blue spaces. Parks were also important for Aurelius, whose map features a church, school and restaurant as out of bounds and shrouded with cloud and rain, compared with the sunshine over Richmond Park, Bishop's Park and Ravenscourt Park (see Figure 4.2; also see the film *My Place, My Space* [2021], co-produced by Stay Home Stories and Write Back, a charity working with young people in the London borough of Barking and Dagenham).

Alongside the importance of being able to see the world beyond the home – and the importance of views of the natural world described by Miriam and Luis – participants also described getting to know and valuing parks and other green spaces more than before. Alexandra, for example, felt 'more ownership of the park',

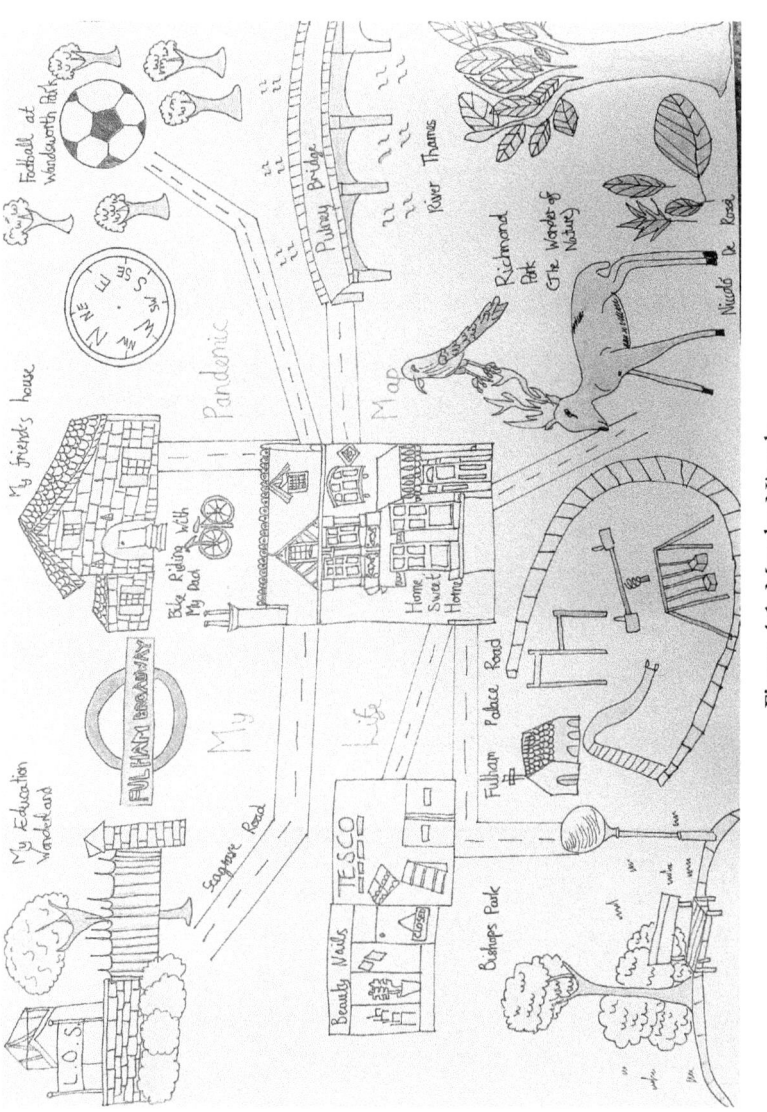

Figure 4.1 Map by Niccolo

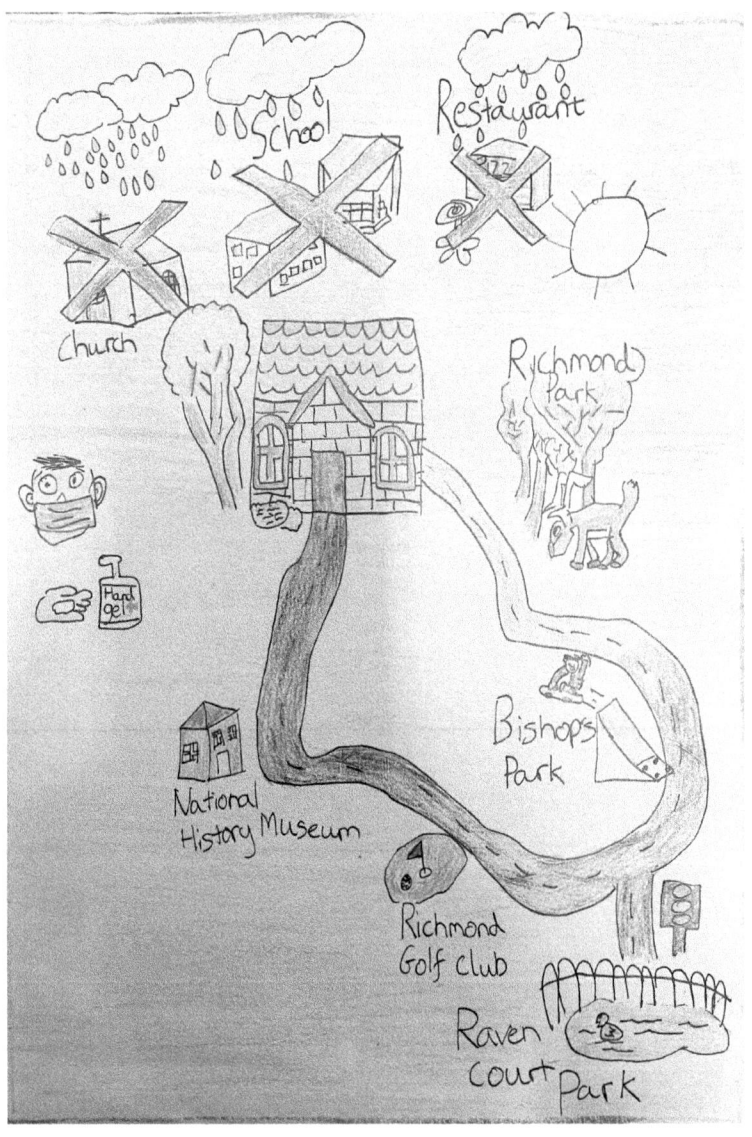

Figure 4.2 Map by Aurelius

while Magda vividly conveyed her deep attachment to Sefton Park in Liverpool through her daily walks:

> I think that I know every nook and cranny of Sefton Park... I became really, really appreciative of that space, and almost kind of started approaching it a little bit more mindfully, I guess, than before. I kind of took it a little bit for granted... I started bird watching in those parks... I've also learned to recognise loads of plants, which I don't think I was able to do before the lockdown... I definitely became mindful of that and I started walking every day.

Our participants – both those with and without access to private or shared gardens – went to parks more frequently and for many reasons: for exercise and fresh air, respite and relaxation, to appreciate nature and for forms of social interaction (also see Burnett et al., 2021). Many, like Em in London, valued visiting parks to pass time, cope with the different pace of life during the pandemic and maintain good mental health:

> I definitely spent a lot of time, a lot, lot, lot more time in my local park. Like there is a whole section of my camera roll which is just filled with images ... just filled with pictures of the wildlife and the skies at different times of day... And actually I do find – I've been looking back through the pictures that I took in the summer lockdown compared to the winter lockdown, and ... charting how the seasons changed throughout the year and ... also my emotions along with it because that November lockdown was like just something else ... that park and those green spaces definitely, definitely became a sanctuary (also see Nightingale et al., 2022 on how artists engaged in new ways with local green spaces).

Yet access to such spaces was far from equal. In the early phases of the pandemic, many parks, such as Victoria Park in east London, were closed because of concerns about social gathering and virus transmission, leaving those without private gardens with limited options to enjoy the supposed benefits of green space. Analysis conducted in London in April 2020 claimed that people in deprived areas and those from BAME backgrounds were negatively and disproportionately affected by these park closures (Duncan et al., 2020). But even when opened, not all groups – including those of certain ages, genders, abilities or who are racially minoritised – could navigate parks and green spaces with ease and without fear of discrimination or hostility (Foster, 2020).

In this section we have focused on the ways in which our participants understood and described their sense of home in relation to a wider sense of dwelling and belonging – or not belonging – in their wider neighbourhood, and the importance of neighbourhood green-blue space in pandemic times. While their insights were mostly positive, experiences during the pandemic raise important questions about spatial inclusion and environmental justice in cities, and especially the future significance of providing green-blue space for human wellbeing (Dobson, 2021). We now turn to the ways in which neighbourly interactions also shaped pandemic experiences of both home and neighbourhood.

Neighbourly interactions

As Sheringham et al. (2023: 722) explain, a wide range of research 'explores "neighbouring" and "neighbourliness" and challenges theories of neighbourhood "disassociation" due to increased privatization and mobility'. This includes analysis of 'the negotiation of privacy and sociability' (Crow et al., 2002: 127); studies on the relative strengths and weaknesses of ties that underpin a sense of community, belonging and/or disaster resilience (Blokland and Nast, 2014; Cheshire, 2015; Felder, 2020; Redshaw and Ingham, 2018); and work on the importance of understanding the sensory dimensions of neighbourly relations (Camilla Lewis, 2020). Building on Sheringham et al.'s (2023) focus on neighbourly encounters within and beyond urban homes and neighbourhoods before the pandemic, we consider the ways in which neighbourly interactions shaped understandings and experiences of pandemic homes and neighbourhoods.

While streets and neighbourhoods felt emptier and more isolated, especially during the first UK lockdown (March–May 2020), our interviews revealed the ways in which neighbourliness itself endured and reshaped. As Leonora from Liverpool told us:

> Gradually, people got, you know, a bit more comfortable popping their heads out ... talking at the doors. I think the closest we came to – everybody came to being near each other was when they were doing the clapping for the NHS when that phase was going on. So, that was a moment where everybody came out to share ... people

were clapping for the NHS, but I think it was also a need for people to see each other and just have that response to each other. You'd see your neighbour across the road, and you'd be, 'Hi'. And waving and smiling. It was so nice to meet someone to smile at and wave to and make that connection, even if it was at a distance because it kind of brought the street alive again, you know, where it's been dead for weeks.

But the possibility for such moments of neighbourly connection depended in part on where people lived. For Luke, also in Liverpool, urban sociality took on a different geography during the pandemic:

[T]he locality itself felt very kind of weirdly isolated. Like all of the back streets that are normally quieter became louder, and our street, which is normally very loud, became really eerie and really deserted. And you couldn't really hear anyone, so that almost felt like a little bit isolating. Like when there was clap[ping] for carers, we couldn't really hear anyone clapping on our street because everyone moved out. But all of the back streets were full of people.

Many interviewees agreed that people had started greeting neighbours more often and appreciating day-to-day social encounters more than before lockdown. For Sheila, for example, who lives in Liverpool,

I do feel that ... I like the neighbourhood, I feel like people do speak to each other more in the streets. And, you know, it's just those chats at, like, supermarkets or the corner shop or just bumping into someone in the street that have changed a bit. And there is sort of, like, a little bit more small talk. Just more saying 'hi', and stuff like that, which definitely wasn't the case before.

Elizabeth, who lives in Finsbury Park in north London where she was born and grew up, also valued seeing and talking to people locally:

The highlight of your day [was] going to the supermarket because then you'd see some people, even though they were all in these masks and you were keeping away from them, it was quite nice. And sometimes you'd ... bump into people and have chats with people in the street that you hadn't spoken to, or people a couple of times came up to me ... and said 'Oh, we used to play with you, we used to play together when we were little'.

Similarly reflecting the importance of shops as places of connection with other people, Em described feeling 'far more acquainted with the local butchers and greengrocers' in her south London neighbourhood and the importance of seeing other people: 'what was really nice as well is seeing people in shops and, even though we weren't necessarily talking, it still felt like some sort of ... a human connection'. This point was echoed by Selin who lives on the Olympic Park in Stratford, east London, and appreciated the open space close to home more than before:

> I don't think previously we would go for a walk in our neighbourhood so much. ... We discovered bits of the neighbourhood that we previously didn't necessarily know about and then started going to those places more often and that has carried on since the lockdown has been eased... We used to take our daughter out for walks and then we ended up actually meeting a lot of people in the neighbourhood ... we kept on running into each other ... meeting new people or running into neighbours that we didn't necessarily know that well. But I think everyone was so eager to connect with each other in the absence of any other sort of social interaction it ... as a neighbourhood we came together quite a bit.

When parks were open, they also served as important public sites of neighbourhood encounter during the pandemic (see Blunt et al., 2022 and Foster, 2020 on park closures during the first lockdown). Even if direct engagement with other people was limited or not allowed, witnessing others dealing with the challenges of restriction and isolation was, for some of our participants, important in validating a sense of the pandemic as a shared experience. New forms of neighbourly interaction became important in helping many people feel more connected with each other during the pandemic through seeing, hearing and talking to each other. Moreover, lockdown and other restrictions meant that for many people, neighbourhood spaces, and particularly parks, enabled them to connect with family members beyond their household or 'bubble'. Saba, for example, spoke about how Sefton Park in Liverpool helped her to stay close to her father, uniting them in new shared daily routines which became vital in later helping her recover from the virus:

> When we were allowed to go for walks with somebody from another household, me and my Dad set up this ... we'd walk round Sefton

Park every day, me and him, and that was brilliant ... because my Dad is staunch, he's like, 'it's just a bit of rain', I would be soaked to the skin, I'd be freezing. And he'd be like, 'you don't have to come love, you don't have to', but then I just knew. And we did it, we did it solid, we did it solid until – and it was mostly because when I got the COVID I got it really bad, it really knocked me for six, it took me quite a while to recover... When it came to ... getting over the COVID and stuff, I wasn't really that strong enough, so he was like, 'come on, let's go to the park'... It was almost like he was trying to help me on my road to recovery and I was also taking it as an opportunity to bond with him as well, so we'd have the best conversations.

As well as family relationships and friendships, the pandemic revealed the importance of neighbourhood relationships and community support. Winne, for example, found that her building's WhatsApp group 'creates a very nice kind of community spirit ... looking after each other or what kind of problems we're encountering'. Julie valued the support of neighbours who delivered food to her doorstep when she was isolating with COVID-19. For some participants who had migrated to London or Liverpool, opportunities for local connection strengthened their sense of the neighbourhood and community as home. As Farah explained, for example,

> I really loved the community around which made me feel like with all the mutual aid things, like neighbours helping each other ... I think that made me feel like ... I do feel like a part of a community, and it does feel like home, and made me also think like home is more like a feeling than like a place.

Community organisations and faith groups played significant roles in providing neighbourly contact and support for local people. Saba, for example, spoke about the role of her Liverpool mosque in keeping people together:

> If a tragedy happens or an adversity happens or something good happens, your faith comes in – kicks in, you know, in one way or another... So the mosque set up a support group to – for all of its congregation in a WhatsApp group so they can keep an eye on each other, they also looked after their neighbours whether they were Muslim or non-Muslim... When COVID happened, because everybody had to pull together, like we knew exactly what the Pakistani community were doing, what the Caribbean community were doing, what that

mosque was doing, what the Somali associations were doing, we all got to hear what was going on in the community... People would go out in the middle of the night to get somebody nappies, you know, or ... our neighbours are all on a WhatsApp group so it was just like somebody needed paracetamol or could somebody pick up an extra bottle of milk, it was – it was so lovely (also see Lawrence et al., 2022 for more on the role of faith groups and leaders during the pandemic).

While community- and faith-led initiatives provided an important source of care and support during the pandemic and helped people to feel anchored in their neighbourhood, they have often developed in the absence of state provision and because of longstanding inequalities that were further deepened during the pandemic. Julie, for example, who volunteered at a food bank in Tower Hamlets throughout the pandemic, described how inadequate state responses to COVID-19 exacerbated existing problems of poverty and austerity:

> Even before the pandemic ... because of austerity and poverty really ... lots of local people have needed the food bank, and that's increased over the pandemic ... and not having resources to support them has meant that they have had to rely on mutual aid and community support ... and I think one of the good things is that we've all found ways to either be supported or support people in our communities whenever there's been need.

While some people talked to their neighbours more than before, others found it hard to do so. Not everyone felt at home in their neighbourhood or that their local urban community was necessarily constructed for, or welcoming of, people like them. Frances, for example, described feeling unable to connect with neighbours, beyond helping one with their internet connection: 'I've been thinking about how, if I hadn't been stuck in my fear, I might have reached out more ... [my] confidence went even lower ... during the pandemic'. As Frances explained, 'I'm still in denial about living here ... and there's always a fear as well about being trans, which is like if you talk to people then they might turn out to be an ally, but they might not and then they'll know too much about you' (see Choi, 2013, on the meaning of home for transgendered people). For Miriam, who felt lonely in her home and neighbourhood in Liverpool,

> I thought that there would be a greater sense of community. But no, there was no communications with neighbours … my neighbours can be … shy or whatever… I say hello, they never say hello back, and that didn't change in lockdown. I thought they would want to create a greater sense of community or at least familiarity, but that didn't happen. So my only contact is with a friend of mine that lives in the building next door, and that didn't change.

While new forms of encounter and conviviality – often on doorsteps or streets close to home, as well as in shops and parks – provided important points of connection for many people, the neighbourhood was hostile and exclusionary for others (see Blunt et al., 2022 for further discussion about the impact of race, ethnicity and immigration status on people during the pandemic). The pandemic took hold in a society where racism was already systemic and heightened racial suspicion and abuse circulated, online and offline. Rogelio, who moved to the UK from the Philippines in 2018, described the 'temporary' nature of London and distinguished between 'home' and a 'dwelling place': '[I]t's a dwelling place. It's not home. It's a dwelling place. It's a provisional space where I can put my body. It's nothing permanent [because of] the dominant culture of disdain for migrants, or suspicion for migrants and people of colour in this country'. He spoke about 'a weird perception that … people of colour are the ones who brought the COVID here', a racialised narrative of contagion and the governance of infectious disease that has deep historical roots (Mallapragada, 2021; White, 2023). Francis was afraid to leave his house because of 'corona racism', and Meilin and Youngsook spoke about anti-Asian sentiment directly, with Meilin recalling a frightening encounter by the canal while out jogging. In Youngsook's words,

> When the pandemic started, apparently, even before the spread in the UK started, there was a huge anti-China, anti-Asian racism. I mean, it was so tense. I experienced it everywhere basically, no one wants to sit next to me. It was really visible, it was [a] subtle but visible kind of aggression everyday (also see Reny and Barreto, 2022; Yunpeng, 2020).

Like Rogelio, Youngsook described London as a 'transitional city', with many residents not in a position to see it as 'their permanent home ground'. While Youngsook felt that she hadn't belonged in London before she moved back to South Korea, she felt more at home once she moved to Hackney on her return, in large part by building a community within the Asian diaspora and with other creative practitioners:

> It creates a sense of home but also it gives you power – it gives you resilience power... You have a power to be resilient against any problems directing to this community. I think that that really helps to build a sense of home or making home ... it's both ways, it's not just inward way, it's also outward way. How can you be strong in who you are and with your culture in this world? ... To be able to be who I am with the non-Asian people, that I want to coexist together, I need to have the strength and resilience.

Neighbourly interactions shaped how our participants felt about their sense of home and belonging both on domestic and neighbourhood scales, with some feeling a greater sense of connectedness than before the pandemic, while others felt increasingly isolated or excluded. The reasons for such differences were attributed to the nature of the neighbourhood, the presence or absence of a sense of community and experiences of racism in a hostile environment, particularly experienced by people of East Asian heritage. In each case, however, people's experiences of home and neighbourhood during the pandemic – whether positive, negative or a mix of the two – were closely bound together.

Conclusion: fairer home-city futures?

While 'stay home' directives in the UK sought to confine people to their homes to limit the spread of COVID-19 and protect the National Health Service (NHS), people's experiences of home during the pandemic were closely shaped by the spaces of the wider neighbourhood, their neighbourly interactions, sense of community and the physical dwelling in which they lived. Rather than seeing home as a fixed and bounded space separate from the neighbourhood, city and world beyond, people's pandemic experiences reveal that, even at its most confined, home is shaped by connections with people beyond the household and places beyond the domestic dwelling. The 'stay home stories' we have discussed in this chapter resonate with wider ideas about 'home-city geographies' (Blunt and Sheringham, 2019) and research undertaken prior to the pandemic on the home as a site of dis/connection within urban neighbourhoods (Sheringham et al., 2023). However, they do so in heightened ways, notably through, first, a new appreciation for, or concern about, the wider neighbourhood, particularly its parks and other green-blue spaces; and, second, more regular encounters and connections with, or a greater sense of disconnection and isolation from, neighbours and local communities.

Our research has demonstrated the deep inequalities that not only shaped people's experiences of, but were also further entrenched by, the COVID-19 pandemic (for further evidence of these inequalities, see Blunt et al., 2022 and Burrell et al., 2021). We end by drawing out some key insights from this chapter and our wider research to inform pandemic recovery agendas on local and national scales that seek to make homes and neighbourhoods fairer and more liveable for all. We recognise that significant structural change, a different political environment and a new vision of cities would be required for these agendas to be fully advanced, but take advantage of the rupture that a global pandemic has brought to imagine a different future.

Our work has shown that understanding people's home lives – and their sense of home beyond as well as within the household and/or domestic dwelling – should be at the heart of future urban place-making and neighbourhood planning. This connects closely with the need to address long-term housing inequality and precarity in the UK in cities like London and Liverpool; and the importance of prioritising adequate space for home-working and access to domestic and/or neighbourhood green space in future housing policies and housing developments. Indeed, the pandemic has emphasised that green spaces are vital for wellbeing, social connection and belonging. Access to such spaces should become more central to policies on physical and mental health, neighbourhood cohesion and children's welfare. This would involve making parks and other green-blue environments safe, welcoming and available to all; and building on improved environmental competencies developed during the COVID-19 pandemic to deepen children's and young people's learning about and appreciation of such local places. The pandemic has also revealed how community, migrant-led and faith organisations can provide vital local support during times of crisis. As cities in the UK recover from the pandemic, there is a need to strengthen coordination, communication and consultation between government and on-the-ground organisations; prioritise core funding for translation services and digital training and access; and create structures within and across community and faith groups to support leaders, particularly those working primarily alone. The possibility of radical change in response to the COVID-19 pandemic feels politically remote, but pandemic experiences of dwelling and belonging on the domestic and neighbourhood scales point to some of the ways that we can all strive to live better locally.

Acknowledgements

The authors acknowledge AHRC funding (AH/V013904/1) for 'Stay Home': Rethinking the Domestic in the COVID-19 Pandemic, funded as part of the UK Research and Innovation (UKRI) rapid response to COVID-19; all of our participants for sharing their experiences of the pandemic; Stay Home Stories community researchers Abigail Agyemang, Yasmin Aktar, Julie Begum, Liza Caruana-Finkel, Filiz Emre, Patrick Graham, Anna Key, Sheekeba Nasimi and Kay Stephens for conducting interviews in London and Liverpool; and editors Frederick Cooper and Des Fitzgerald for their very helpful feedback on this chapter.

Note

1 We use 'neighbourhood' to refer to the places local to where people live and with which they identify. This could be a specific physical space or administratively defined place but might also be an 'imagined' space; we are interested in people's pandemic *sense* of place and its relationship to their ideas of home.

References

Alonso, Lucia and Jacoby, Sam (2023), The impact of housing design and quality on wellbeing: Lived experiences of the home during COVID-19 in London. *Cities & Health*, 7(4), 615–627. doi:10.1080/23748834.2022.2103391

Aznar, Ana, et al. (2021), Home-schooling during COVID-19 lockdown: Effects of coping style, home space and everyday creativity on stress and home-schooling outcomes. *Couple and Family Psychology: Research and Practice*, 10(4), 294–312.

Baxter, Richard and Brickell, Katherine (2014), For home *un*making. *Home Cultures*, 11(2), 133–143.

Blokland, Talja and Nast, Julia (2014), From public familiarity to comfort zone: The relevance of absent ties for belonging in Berlin's mixed neighbourhoods. *International Journal of Urban and Regional Research*, 38(4), 1142–1159.

Blunt, Alison and Bonnerjee, Jayani (2013), Home, city and diaspora: Anglo-Indian and Chinese attachments to Calcutta. *Global Networks*, 13(2), 220–240.

Blunt, Alison and Sheringham, Olivia (2019), Home-city geographies: Urban dwelling and mobility. *Progress in Human Geography*, 43(5), 815–834.

Blunt, Alison, Ebbensgaard, Casper Laing and Sheringham, Olivia (2020), The 'living of time': Entangled temporalities of home and the city. *Transactions of the Institute of British Geographers*, 46(1). doi: 10.1111/tran.12405

Blunt, Alison and Dowling, Robyn (2022), *Home*, 2nd edn. Abingdon: Routledge.

Blunt, Alison, et al. (2022), *At Home in London during COVID-19: Policy Recommendations and Key Findings*. London: Queen Mary University of London. Available at: http://stayhomestories.co.uk/london-report

Bonnerjee, Jayani (2012), Dias-para: Neighbourhood, memory and the city. *South Asian Diaspora*, 4(1), 5–25.

Bower, Marlee, Buckle, Caitlin, Rugel, Emily, et al. (2023), 'Trapped', 'anxious', and 'traumatised': COVID-19 intensified the impact of housing inequality on Australians' mental health. *International Journal of Housing Policy*, 23(2), 260–291. doi: 10.1080/19491247.2021.1940686

Bryson, John, Andres, Lauren and Davies, Andrew (2020), COVID-19, virtual Church services and a new temporary geography of home. *Tijdschrift voor economische en sociale geografie*, 111(3), 360–372. doi: 10.1111/tesg.12436

Burnett, Hannah, et al. (2021), Change in time spent visiting and experiences of green space following restrictions on movement during the COVID-19 pandemic: A nationally representative, cross-sectional study of UK adults. *BMJ Open*, 11(3).

Burrell, Kathy (2014), Spilling over from the street: Contextualizing domestic space in an inner-city neighbourhood. *Home Cultures*, 11(2), 145–166.
Burrell, Kathy, et al. (2021), *At Home in Liverpool during COVID-19*. London: Queen Mary University of London. Available at: https://stayhomestories.co.uk/liverpool-report
Cheshire, Lynda (2015), 'Know your neighbours': Disaster resilience and the normative practices of neighbouring in an urban context. *Environment & Planning A*, 47(5), 1081–1099.
Cheshire, Lynda, Easthope, Hazel and ten Have, Charlotte (2021), Unneighbourliness and the unmaking of home. *Housing, Theory and Society*, 38(2), 133–151. doi: 10.1080/14036096.2019.1705384
Choi, Youngsook (2013), 'The Meaning of Home for Transgendered People' in Yvette Taylor and Michelle Addison (eds), *Queer Presences and Absences*. Basingstoke: Palgrave Macmillan, pp. 118–140.
Crow, Graham, Allan, Graham and Summers, Marcia (2002), Neither busybodies nor nobodies: Managing proximity and distance in neighbourly relations. *Sociology*, 36(1), 127–145.
Dimopoulos, Kostas, Koutsampelas, Christos and Tsatsaroni, Anna (2021), Home schooling through online teaching in the era of COVID-19: Exploring the role of home-related factors that deepen educational inequalities across European societies. *European Educational Research Journal*, 20(4), 479–497.
Dobson, Julian (2021), Wellbeing and blue-green space in post-pandemic cities: Drivers, debates and departures. *Geography Compass*, 15(10), 1–15.
Duncan, Pamela, MacIntyre, Niamh and Cutler, Sam (2020), Coronavirus park closures hit BAME and poor Londoners most. *Guardian*, 10 April.
Erfani, Goran and Bahrami, Bakhtiar (2023), COVID and the home: The emergence of new urban life practised under pandemic-imposed restrictions. *Cities & Health*, 7(4), 548–555. doi: 10.1080/23748834.2022.2029241
Felder, Maxime (2020), Strong, weak and invisible ties: A relational perspective on urban coexistence. *Sociology*, 54(4), 675–692.
Fitzgerald, Des (2020), Stay the fuck at home. Somatosphere, 13 April. Available at http://somatosphere.net/2020/stay-the-fuck-at-home.html/
Foster, Dawn (2020), The sinister new politics of public space: Your prejudice is showing. *Huck*, 6 April. Available at: www.huckmag.com/perspectives/opinion-perspectives/the-sinister-new-politics-of-public-space/
Grewal, Kiran, et al., eds. (2020), Confronting 'the household'. Feminist Review, web log series, 26 May. Available at: https://femrev.wordpress.com/2020/05/26/confronting-the-household
Institute for Government. (2022), Timeline of UK government coronavirus lockdowns and restrictions. Available at: www.instituteforgovernment.org.uk/charts/uk-government-coronavirus-lockdowns

Islam, Asiya (2022), Work-from/at/for-home: CoVID-19 and the future of work – a critical review. *Geoforum*, 128, 33–36.

Lawrence, Miri, Owens, Alastair and Blunt, Alison (2022), *Home, Faith and COVID-19: Insights from the Pandemic and Opportunities for the Future*. London: Queen Mary University of London. Available at: www.stayhomestories.co.uk/faith-resource-guide

Lewis, Camilla (2020), Listening to community: The aural dimensions of neighbouring. *The Sociological Review*, 68(1), 94–109.

Lewis, Sophie (2020), The coronavirus crisis shows it's time to abolish the family, Open Democracy, 24 March. Available at: www.opendemocracy.net/en/oureconomy/coronavirus-crisis-shows-its-time-abolish-family/

Maalsen, Sophia and Dowling, Robyn (2020), Covid-19 and the accelerating smart home. *Big Data & Society*, July–December, 1–5. doi: 10.1177/2053951720938073

Mallapragada, Madhavi (2021), Asian Americans as racial contagion. *Cultural Studies*, 35(2–3), 279–290.

Mehta, Vikas (2020), The new proxemics: COVID-19, social distancing, and sociable space, *Journal of Urban Design*, 25(6), 669–674.

Mell, Ian and Whitten, Meredith (2021), Access to nature in a post COVID-19 world: Opportunities for green infrastructure financing, distribution and equitability in urban planning. *International Journal of Environmental Research and Public Health*, 18, 1–16.

Nightingale, Eithne, Blunt, Alison and Owens, Alastair (2022), *Artists, Other Creative Practitioners and COVID-19: Personal Experiences and Policy Insights*. London: Queen Mary University of London. Available at: www.stayhomestories.co.uk/art-report

Ottoni, Callista, Winters, Meghan and Sims-Gould, Joanie (2022), 'We see each other from a distance': Neighbourhood social relationships during the COVID-19 pandemic matter for older adults' social connectedness. *Health & Place*, 76. doi: 10.1016/j.healthplace.2022.102844

Pandey, Kritika, Parreñas, Rhacel Salazar and Sabio, Gianne Sheena (2021), Essential and expendable: Migrant domestic workers and the COVID-19 pandemic. *American Behavioral Scientist*, 65(10), 1287–1301.

Piquero, Alex, et al. (2021), Domestic violence during the COVID-19 pandemic: Evidence from a systematic review and meta-analysis. *Journal of Criminal Justice*, 74. doi: 10.1016/j.jcrimjus.2021.101806

Preece, Jenny, McKee, Kim, Robinson, David, et al. (2023), Urban rhythms in a small home: COVID-19 as a mechanism of exception. *Urban Studies*, 60(9), 1650–1667. doi: 10.1177/00420980211018136

Rao, Smriti, et al. (2021), Human mobility, COVID-19, and policy responses: The rights and claims-making of migrant domestic workers. *Feminist Economics*, 27(1–2), 254–270.

Redshaw, Sarah and Ingham, Valerie (2018), 'Neighbourhood is if they come out and talk to you': Neighbourhood connections and bonding social capital. *Sociology*, 54(4), 557–573.

Reny, Tyler T. and Barreto, Matt A. (2022), Xenophobia in the time of pandemic: Othering, anti-Asian attitudes and COVID-19. *Politics, Groups and Identities*, 10(2), 209–232.

Sheringham, Olivia, Ebbensgaard, Casper Laing and Blunt, Alison (2023), 'Tales from other people's houses': Home and dis/connection in an East London neighbourhood. *Social & Cultural Geography*, 24(5), 719–734. doi: 10.1080/14649365.2021.1965197

Trasberg, Terje and Cheshire, James (2023), Spatial and social disparities in the decline of activities during the COVID-19 lockdown in Greater London. *Urban Studies*, 60(8), 1427–1447. doi: 10.1177/00420980211040409

Vertovec, Steven, ed. (2015), *Diversities Old and New: Migration and Socio-Spatial Patterns in New York, Singapore and Johannesburg*. Basingstoke: Palgrave Macmillan.

Waldron, Richard (2023), Experiencing housing precarity in the private rental sector during the covid-19 pandemic: The case of Ireland. *Housing Studies*, 38(1), 84–106. doi:10.1080/02673037.2022.2032613

White, Alexandre (2023), *Epidemic Orientalism: Race, Capital and the Governance of Infectious Disease*. Stanford, CA: Stanford University Press.

Women's Aid. (2020), *A Perfect Storm: The Impact of the Covid-19 Pandemic on Domestic Abuse Survivors and the Services Supporting Them*. Bristol: Women's Aid. Available at: www.womensaid.org.uk/a-perfect-storm-the-impact-of-the-covid-19-pandemic-on-domestic-abuse-survivors-and-the-services-supporting-them.

Yunpeng, Du (Dery) (2020), Go home: Coronavirus, national protection, and the last path towards home, Disruptive Inequalities. Available at: https://disruptiveinequalities.com/2020/08/03/the-lost-path-towards-home

5

Crisis and engagement: The emotional toll of museum work during the COVID-19 pandemic

Elizabeth Crooke and David Farrell-Banks

As locations that interpret and present the histories of places and people, museums are affective spaces with emotional impacts shaping how we think about ourselves and others. Flora Kaplan's book *Museums and the Making of 'Ourselves'* is a reminder that museums are about us, and when our stories are told in museum spaces those stories will affect us (Kaplan, 1994). In *Museums, Emotion and Memory Culture*, Gönül Bozoğlu details her own emotional responses to her research field notes, becoming an increasingly central part of her work (Bozoğlu, 2019). The emotional impact of museums is primarily considered from the perspective of the visitor, with museums as 'places where people go to feel, to be emotional' (Smith, 2014: 125). What is less well established is the emotional resonance of museums as a place of work. Those employed in museums, cultural or heritage sectors can become rooted in their work, drawing upon their personal histories as motivation and inspiration, influencing the subject matter they engage with or the approaches they take. For instance, the notion of the 'activist curator' is now well established as an alignment of personal values and workplace roles (Hollows, 2019). Taken together, these examples demonstrate that the outcome of work can be as personally meaningful as it is professionally important. In the context of the COVID-19 pandemic, we found that the emotional labour of museum work was both exposed and intensified in workers' responses to the crisis.

This chapter is a consideration of the impact of the COVID-19 pandemic on the museum workforce in Northern Ireland, drawing upon findings from the UKRI-funded project Museums, Crisis and Covid19, based at Ulster University. With the Museums

Association, the National Lottery Heritage Fund, Northern Ireland Museums Council and the Tower Museum Derry/Londonderry, the project worked alongside the museum sector as it adapted and moved online; advised on the importance of financial support measures that proved a lifeline for the sector; and explored how museums re-articulated their roles during the pandemic. With the principal outputs focusing on changes to museum operations, digital adaptations and the wellbeing role of the museum sector, this chapter focuses on findings beyond the scope of the original project (Crooke et al., 2022a; 2022b; 2022c). While undertaking interviews and focus groups with staff in museums, documenting the impact of the public health measures on the sector, the researchers had not predicted quite how much our contributors would reveal about how the pandemic altered their relationship with their work.[1] As well as changes to routine, methods of working and concerns about precarity, which are shared by other sectors, we found impacts arising from being *museum* workers. The idea of the museum community changed, both in terms of how staff connected with their audiences and the experiences of community among those who work in museums. As researchers, we learned about the emotional toll of leaving the museum and returning. Individuals spoke about the personal impacts of needing to halt or transform methods of public engagement and outreach work, knowing that some users depended on museum programmes for social interaction. Additionally, respondents voiced the added uncertainty of working in a sector that appeared to have become even more vulnerable, given that most museums relied, at that time, on visitors to the physical building. Here the emotional toll is pushed even further. Knowing the challenges of public and third-sector funding, museum workers needed not only to be relevant and resilient during the crisis, but also to be seen to be making those adaptations by those responsible for allocating public funds to the sector.

During our engagements with museum staff, the importance of their work and the personal connections with it was a re-occurring theme. We found that the pandemic both exposed and intensified how personally meaningful and emotionally affecting museum work was. Our sample of interviewees represented museum management, curatorial and front-of-house work: roles were critical to the original Museums, Crisis and Covid19 project, which focused specifically on museum-based tasks of collections care, museum interpretation and digital adaptation in accredited museums. During the years of museum closures and re-openings, the significance of established museum tasks such as collecting, display and outreach work changed. Rapid-response collecting added emotional weight because the museum staff undertaking that role were equally vested in the pandemic experience, while carrying a sense of collective responsibility to document the pandemic for future museum audiences. The greater dependency on digital platforms during the pandemic brought with it reflection upon how to re-create an emotional engagement with the past at a physical remove. Curators and education staff in the sector referred to a professional sense of duty to collect stories and objects that would document the impact of the pandemic and represent it to future generations. As one of our contributors put it, 'we knew we were living through something very big and, given the museum's social role, we felt a responsibility to collect at a time of crisis' (Brownlee, 20 October 2021).

This chapter demonstrates how deeply personal and emotionally affecting museum work can be, and how that was heightened during the pandemic. Our goal is to explore what this disruption revealed about how museum workers, who engaged with our project, strategically identified with their work and how that shaped their practice. We suggest that focusing on the workplace is another route to understanding museum impacts, purposes, value and ethics, an avenue that is barely touched on in existing museum studies literature (Black, 2021; Macdonald, 2006; Marstine, 2011). By drawing upon interviews, focus group discussions and workshops with people working in and with museums, from a variety of positions and institutions in Northern Ireland, this chapter begins to fill that gap in our understanding. In the discussion that follows, we focus on the personal and emotional impacts of COVID-19 on museum staff and their practice across three areas. First, we provide an account of the COVID-19 crisis as experienced by the museum sector and what it reveals about how museum workers navigate and articulate museum purposes. We then move to a consideration of the idea of 'career shock' (Akkermans et al., 2020; Hite and McDonald, 2020), and the impact of this on sector resilience and wellbeing – again looking at this from the perspective of reimagining museum purposes. Finally, building on these foundations, we move to an exploration of the emotional labour and emotion work connected to working through the pandemic.

Museums, Crisis and Covid19: rethinking purposes

Crisis is a term that has potentially suffered from overuse (Deans, 2022), often utilised to capture attention but with little critical engagement given to its use (Graf and Jarausch, 2017, cited in Deans, 2022). Friel and Beavis described the pandemic as 'an acute, sudden, and unexpected crisis that was expected to be short-term in duration'; it then 'quickly evolved into a chronic, unpredictable and unprecedented global life-threatening episode' (2022: 16). For many, 'crisis' became the prevailing understanding of the pandemic: nationally and internationally, the museum sector wrote about the period as one of crisis (Agostino et al., 2020; Christiansen, 2020; Potts, 2020), and the word was used by our interviewees both in our conversations and publication (such as Blair, 2021). For our purposes, we utilise the affordances of crisis to communicate 'multiple senses that things have gone wrong' (Whitehead et al., 2019: 2), for many groups and generations at once, precipitating 'changes, vulnerabilities, reorganisations, and new life structures' (Moura et al., 2021: 376). In the context of COVID-19, there is a constructive flexibility within this understanding of crisis that opens our view to the multiple, differing experiences of the COVID-19 pandemic from one person to the next, as well as the shifting nature of different phases of the pandemic. The experience of a crisis from within, as we will explore further below, comes with an understanding that there was a time prior to this crisis emerging, and there will be a time after it has passed (Whitehead et al., 2019). This draws attention to the temporal boundaries imposed on crises as events. As with any understanding of an 'event', however, these boundaries are selective (see Farrell-Banks, 2023; Wagner-Pacifici, 2021). The beginnings and ends of the pandemic, whether understood as crisis, event or by some other conceptualisation, are and will be socially constructed. It is evident to us that there is some uncertainly about when the COVID-19 crisis will come to an 'end', particularly given that the legacy of COVID-19 is likely to merge with other societal challenges such as the cost-of-living crisis and the effects of climate change.

The impacts of COVID-19 and associated protective measures such as periods of restriction on movement, gatherings and business operations, have also exacerbated pre-existing inequalities both nationally and globally (Bajos et al., 2021; Perry et al., 2021). At points of crisis, however, positive and negative emotions can co-mingle and change (Slaughter et al., 2021). Anxiety over the impacts of the pandemic, for example, might be felt alongside relief that measures were being taken to combat the virus. Subsequent periods of restriction may have been met with frustration or a sense of fatigue as the pandemic moved into a second year. Within the United Kingdom, restrictions have been seen to negatively impact the mental health of those groups already likely to experience relatively poor mental health prior to the outbreak of COVID-19 (Blundell et al., 2022). We can also expect that museum staff and audiences were impacted to differing degrees by the pandemic, in terms of their job security, family stability and impacts upon mental health. The vulnerabilities felt and the social impacts that emerge from the pandemic and the public health response to it will be uneven depending on dimensions such as class, gender and ethnicity (Moura et al., 2021; Zhou and Kan, 2021). While the remainder of this chapter is focused upon the experiences of museums and their staff, each of these experiences sits within this broad context.

Museums, Crisis and Covid19 found that the organisational health of a museum going into the pandemic shaped how the institution addressed the challenges posed by closure, loss of income and staffing changes (Crooke et al., 2022a). How museum management teams handled the crisis, both in relation to staff management, as well as the connection with audiences, will have longer-term impacts on the dynamics within and outside museums. In our discussion with museum staff regarding their experiences of furlough, communication between management and the staff likely to be placed on furlough was key to shaping both the anticipation and implementation of the scheme. The Director of Operations at National Museums Northern Ireland told us that, at the outset, staff saw the scheme as 'tantamount to redundancy', whereas the senior management saw it as a temporary measure 'safeguarding the future of the organisation' and, it was hoped, protecting against the need for redundancies (Catney, 1 March 2021). Across local and independent museums, the experience of furlough varied: some staff remained working throughout the pandemic, while others came on and off furlough. In smaller museums that might only operate with four or five full-time staff, the museum curator/manager remained in post, overseeing other staff taking periods of furlough during pandemic phases. In a museum within a Local Authority, all staff took their 'turn' at going on furlough. A museum worker described her managers as handling the scheme 'efficiently and sensitively'. Nevertheless, the longer a person had been on furlough, 'people started to feel a bit like they didn't have a purpose or a role' and 'that got a few people down' (Anon_07). In the first year of the pandemic, it was estimated that two-thirds of those working in museums were in vulnerable roles – many of which were audience-facing roles, rather than management or curatorial roles (Johnston et al., 2020: 4). A crystallising statement during our project interviews occurred when a manager in the museum/heritage sector referred to the visitor team as 'low hanging fruit', because they would be the first in line to be put on furlough, revealing the uneven vulnerabilities among museum staff (Anon_09).

The pandemic drew attention to a subset of positions within the museum sector that are more precarious than other roles. This inequality within the museum workforce pre-dates the pandemic. Workforce campaigns, led by the Museums Association and the grassroots body Fair Museum Jobs, have demonstrated that those in front-of-house positions experience less agency and opportunity in their roles (Fair Museum Jobs, 2020; Museums Association, 2022a). Furthermore, at a Future Museum Policy: Northern Ireland event (Ulster University, September 2022), a point was made about the lack of voice among front-of-house or lower-pay-grade museum staff in discussions regarding museums policy for Northern Ireland. This comment from a museum worker suggests that those most vulnerable during the pandemic continue to feel excluded from the conversations that directly impact their future. While there is often a shared vocational commitment across different forms of work within the museum sector, it remains the case that some workers will operate in a significantly more precarious position while also having fewer opportunities to voice their opinions on the sector's future.

Career shock, career resilience and wellbeing in museums

In the past two decades, museums have focused increasingly on their caring role for audiences (Morse, 2021); in direct reference to that practice, in 2022, the UK Museums Association asked its members to 'mirror their commitments and actions to support wellbeing in their communities and support the wellbeing of those that work in and with their museum' (Museums Association, 2022b: n.p.). Recognition of the growing pressures of working in the sector is evident in the Museums Association's campaigns for fair working conditions for those working in and with museums. During the pandemic, a particular focus on the mental health of museum sector staff led to the establishment of an online Wellbeing Hub still accessible in 2023. The need for such an intervention recognised that working from home and furlough created disconnection and loneliness, impacting both professional and personal wellbeing (Museums Association, 2022b). As the pandemic progressed, the Museums Association added further resources on the theme of 'understanding your emotions'. Recognising the connections between 'logical thinking and emotional reflection', this material was directly speaking to the impact of responses to the pandemic and offered methods for navigating furlough, returning to work or handling any risk of redundancy (Museums Association, 2022b). Here we find national recognition that occupational health is a risk factor for the sector where employment can be precarious, contract-based and low paid – all issues aggravated by the pandemic.

During the pandemic, it was impossible to separate lived experiences of COVID-19 from concerns in the workplace. Evident among museum staff were emotions such as grief, disgust, anger and fear, exacerbated by social, political and medical uncertainties (Stanley et al., 2021). Museum workers were navigating personal experiences and concerns, while transforming a museum service which they hoped would still be relevant to their audiences. In the opening months of the pandemic, and the first imposition of significant social restrictions in March 2020, feelings of fear and anxiety were understandable. In his interview a year after the first lockdown, Michael Fryer, Outreach Officer at Northern Ireland War Memorial, said 'I remember how strange it was, just the feeling of something was happening or the sense of foreboding' (Fryer, 30

April 2021). Speaking early in the pandemic, a manager working in a museum within a Local Authority described her thoughts when the museum had just closed for the first 'lockdown'. Sitting at home, about to go into Zoom meeting, she was thinking, 'My God, how am I going to manage these people remotely?'; and, because a furlough scheme had not yet been announced, 'How do I keep these people employed' (Anon_05). In a second interview some months later, she reflected that 'I felt I had an awful responsibility in the sense of… I think you need to take yourself back to the mindset at the time. People were frightened and they didn't know what was happening' (Anon_05).

Emerging from human resources literature is the narrative of both the pandemic as a 'crisis' and a 'career shock', the latter explained as a 'disruptive and extraordinary event' outside an individual's control (Akkermans et al., 2020: 1). Such an event has an impact on a person's career, determining 'what types of jobs will thrive, survive or become obsolete' (Hite and McDonald, 2020: 478). Hite and McDonald suggest that career resilience is shaped both by individual characteristics and contextual factors: the former focusing on individual traits such as skills, attitudes and behaviours; and the latter being an outcome of workplace support, job characteristics and effective networks. Hite and McDonald suggest that this combination determines ways in which an individual or institution assesses a situation and adapts for more positive outcomes. If this twofold explanation of resilience is taken as a guide, it is essential to recognise that the workplace context is a factor in individual agency. The 'career shock' of museum closures meant that staff had to navigate the experience of furlough and job insecurity and, when they returned to work, adapt their roles. Systematic inequalities in workplaces have been to the detriment of personal agency, a point highlighted by the Museums Association workforce campaigns. This very factor was critical to workforce experiences of the pandemic, which varied greatly among the diversity of roles in the museum sector.

Because our sample of interviewees were people hoping for a lifetime of work in the museum or heritage sectors, the notion of career shock is reflected in how they described the impact of the pandemic on their working practices. In our project interviews with museum managers, the experience of shock is evident in the language they use to describe the realisation that the pandemic was leading to museum closures and radically different ways of working. One referred to it as 'an out-of-ordinary event' (Anon_01), implying it was something no one could plan for; another described it as 'unprecedented', and a time 'when everything went pear shaped' (Anon_05). The lack of institutional preparedness for such an event is a damning reflection of governmental communication and action in response to their own guidelines. In 2017, the *National Risk Register of Civil Emergencies* advised that 'there is a high probability of a flu pandemic occurring' (Cabinet Office, 2017: 34). Despite warnings to government from the public health sectors that a pandemic was only a matter of time, preparedness for such an event was severely lacking when it arrived (Mellish et al., 2020). Leading up to the first lockdown, a staff member working in an independent museum described the time as 'so stressful ... it was quite chaotic ... it was kind of frustrating ... it was difficult for you to plan' (Anon_07).

The impact of this career shock emerged in our interviews with furloughed museum staff, although not always in the manner that we might have expected. A member of front-of-house museum staff said that while 'it was difficult not working [...] I was getting paid to not work. I could have been out of a job' (Anon_08). For this individual, it was the relief that furlough support had been provided that initiated a strong emotional response. To be furloughed was far more welcome than being made redundant – the outcome for hundreds of staff in the wider heritage sector, such as the National Trust (2020). Our interviewee told us that 'Overall, I did count myself just so lucky – sorry, I'm getting emotional – to be in the position of being eligible for furlough'. With a slight pause to hold off tears, the interview itself seemed to provide a release of emotion as the experience of furlough was relived. This emotion returned when the re-opening of museums was discussed: 'For those of us that were on furlough, it was so nice getting back into the museum – I'm getting emotional again' (Anon_08). In both cases, the most emotional point in the interview came when discussing experiences of relief – a relief at being provided some job security through furlough, and later, a relief at being back to work.

For those working in museums, career resilience is often tied to the larger issue of sector resilience – keeping museums relevant and in demand. Across the sector, museum institutions and individual staff embraced the need to change their programming and delivery during the pandemic, both to serve what audiences needed and as a protective measure. A manager of a museum within a Local Authority described the opening months of social restrictions and enforced museum closures as a 'steep learning curve' (Anon_02). Those who were able to adapt to the challenges of the pandemic, whether that was navigation of the furlough scheme, or adapting their work when back in the museum, found personal satisfaction from that. Curator Manager Heather McGuicken, of North Down Museum, was one of a number of museum workers who saw the museum closures as bringing a rare opportunity to return to reflect and take stock, saying, 'that part of it was actually great. Very therapeutic' (McGuicken, 23 March 2021). A curator at an independent museum shared the value of being able to get to the museum while it was closed, to escape the reality of the health concerns during the pandemic. While respecting social distancing, she and a colleague worked in the museum stores one day a week, both checking collections and recording content for social media. She described those regular visits to the collection as important from 'a wellbeing perspective', adding, 'It has actually helped us – the staff – to purposely take one day and go in and work in the museum and try to do these [social media] projects. The projects have actually helped the staff's confidence, the staff's mental wellbeing' (Anon_03). Weathering the pandemic, learning new skills and involvement in pandemic-related work demonstrated a resilience that has given some in the sector confidence moving forward.

The changes that museum staff have embraced, if maintained, have potential to completely change the reach and positioning of regional museums. A curator at National Museums Northern Ireland reflected on the impact of embracing digital media. Before 2020, the digital offering – of virtual exhibitions, podcasts and meetings via digital platforms – was minimal. Now, connectivity has 'moved us forward ... it's really accelerated that process' (Anon_06). Thinking back over the international meetings and events hosted via Zoom, she suggests that the pandemic transformed how she and her colleagues thought about their museum service. She explained that greater connectivity, enabled by the digital transformation, has given staff 'renewed energy' to adapt how they engage with audiences (Anon_06). Some museum staff in the field found that new learning and opportunities for reflection on museum practice during the pandemic have been positive. The pandemic had 'given us the permission to do things that we hadn't done before' (Anon_05). For another interviewee, this had been a process of embracing new forms of communication, describing the pandemic as having 'definitely opened opportunities for us' (Anon_02).

Across the board, those we interviewed took pride in how they adapted during the pandemic – whether that was learning new digital skills, adapting museum programming and connecting with museum professionals in new online forms. This is best represented by a statement from Michael Fryer at Northern Ireland War Memorial: 'It's certainly challenged me, but I think challenged me in a good way' (Fryer, 30 April 2021). Another interviewee reported that furlough brought some breathing space to reflect on career objectives: 'I was able to use that in thinking about what I wanted to do and how I could show the evidence that I was able to do that'. This interviewee was particularly proud that 'despite everything over the last year and a half with Covid, the project still was meeting its objectives … we were really proud of that' (Anon_07). Here we see the demonstration of career resilience as a valuable experience. Both interviewees described the confidence they now had for facing future challenges; it is evident, however, that confidence alone does not enable individuals and teams to overcome challenges. Rather, combinations of financial, training and welfare support as well as clear communication from senior management were critical to good outcomes, and experiences of this varied across the sector. For instance, museum staff working in our sample of independent museums found themselves well-supported in exploring new ways of engaging audiences during museum closures, whereas staff in some Local Authority museums found themselves re-deployed to other areas of Local Authority work, taking them away from core museum roles.

The disruptions precipitated by the public health response to the pandemic have changed how museum workers think both emotionally and strategically about their place of work. When people returned from furlough, and found they could still provide a relevant service despite the challenges of the pandemic, this was both personally satisfying and reinforced the societal relevance of the institution within which individuals worked. For staff working in front-of-house, learning and outreach roles, audience relevance was key. Greatest work satisfaction was found among museum staff when management demonstrated both an understanding of and support for adapting these roles to the needs of audiences during the pandemic.

Emotion work and emotional labour

In the past decade, due to an increasing focus within heritage and museum studies on how audiences interact with the past, scholars better understand the affective and emotional capacities of museums and heritage sites. Research has drawn attention to how objects, buildings, exhibitions and texts can elicit a felt response in those interacting with them (Bozoğlu, 2019; McCreanor et al., 2019; Smith, 2020; Smith et al., 2018; Tolia-Kelly et al., 2017; Witcomb, 2015). We can think of museums as spaces filled with 'objects bearing information and transmitting emotions'; they are places of 'memory and knowledge', encouraging people to 'view, contemplate and connect' (Sandahl, 2019: 6). Across museums, curatorial teams and collaborators work on exhibitions and programmes that are often emotionally affecting. Of the staff we interviewed, some had experience of representing the Northern Ireland conflict and its legacy in museum spaces, an area of work that is shaped by individual and lived experiences of the past four decades, as well as professional demands (Crooke, 2021; 2024). Consequently, museum outreach and engagement staff working on projects around memory and reminiscence often find themselves dealing with topics both personally and collectively affecting. Furthermore, the daily interactions of front-of-house staff represent the emotional labour inherent to any public-facing role. Museums are institutions which, with a background in communicating power (Bennett, 1995) and communicating with a degree of authority (Smith, 2006), can also impact how we feel within these spaces. In other words, we are all likely to have an idea of how we think we should behave within a museum.

This turn towards a focus on affect and emotion in museum studies recognises that emotional engagement with museums is an 'inevitable and foundational' component of their practice (Bozoğlu, 2019: 8). Hollows (2019), for example, sees increasing alignment of personal and work identities among museum staff working in community-facing roles. Based on interviews with museum staff, she found that those who embraced social justice roles welcomed value placed on both the *emotional* and the *technical* aspects of that work. Ealasaid Munro (2014) describes museums as places full of emotion, found in paying closer attention to the degree to which museum displays can create an emotional response. Andrea Witcomb (2015) introduced the concept of a 'pedagogy of feeling', directing attention to the way in which exhibits can be staged to encourage a particular 'affective encounter' from the visitor. Munro (2014) reflects on community engagement practice in Glasgow Museums where the museum was offered as a 'safe, supportive space' where people could 'learn from and make sense of past experience ... [and] build resilience', thus 'contributing to individuals' emotional wellbeing' (2014: 47). We could, therefore, view emotional engagement with museums not only as inevitable and foundational, but also designable.

The recognition of the emotional capacity of interactions with museum exhibits can inform practice within the museum, both as a workplace and a public space, as we move through the pandemic and start to respond to its lasting effects. The moments at which a strong emotional response to experiences of the pandemic might emerge can be unexpected, and an awareness of this will have to feed into the development of exhibitions that respond to the pandemic itself. The pandemic also prompts a shift in our view of experiences of emotional labour. Arlie Russell Hochschild coined the term 'emotional labour' to refer to the management of emotions required within public-facing wage-labour, which can be to the expense of a worker's wellbeing (Hochschild, 1983). Public-facing museum roles fit this description, with staff expected to engage with the public in a friendly, welcoming manner. In the interview above, however, we see emotional labour coalesced with personal emotional responses coming with a return to work. This, too, comes alongside a need to engage in emotion work. 'Emotion work', as distinct from emotional labour, is work focused on 'dealing with other people's emotions' (Dickson-Swift et al., 2009: 62). This emotion work now includes a need to be conscious of the feelings that come with a return to in-person museum activity during a pandemic that is, at the time of writing in late 2022, ongoing; even if social restrictions have been removed. The emotional labour of the workplace can materialise in a mix of relief, anxiety, fear and hope, within both staff and visitors. The additional toll that this emotional labour may take on workers in public-facing roles, particularly in spaces that were subject to long enforced closures, might not yet be fully realised.

The tendency for those in the sector to find themselves personally rooted in their work is informed by the nature of the task and is one that is rarely interrogated by the sector. The methods used by museum professionals, such as outreach community work, demand that museum staff get close to and engaged with their users. In addition, the very materiality of museum work, when it includes collections or themes associated with difficult and sensitive subjects, is emotionally affecting. The pandemic placed an increasing demand on museum staff to reach out to those isolated due to lockdowns or clinical vulnerability. Combining workplace changes with an increasing need for socially engaged museum work suggests a doubling up of the emotional toll of the pandemic on the sector.

Museum staff felt a duty and responsibility to record this extraordinary time; curators referred to their responsibility for collecting the pandemic, which in some cases was cathartic for both museum staff and those generating the materials. At the Irish Linen Centre & Lisburn Museum (ILCLM), the Covid-19 and Me project brought together stories, memories, photographs, videos and audio files that captured audiences' experiences of the pandemic. Inspired by established outreach programmes, audiences were posed two provocations: 'What stories or lessons do you think future generations should take from the pandemic?', and 'A hundred years from now people will want to know what happened, how we experienced and dealt with the pandemic' (ILCLM, 2020). The museum sought to enhance participation and interaction when people may have been fearful or lonely. Working with audiences, the museum introduced the method of life-writing, aware that to write can be cathartic even for traumatic experiences. The museum encouraged individuals to describe their situation, asking the following questions: 'Do you do things differently now?', 'Is communication different?', 'How do you feel about social isolation?'

and 'Is there something that has made you happy or encouraged you to be positive during the present situation?' (ILCLM, 2020).

At a time of increased emotional uncertainty and pressure, social distancing measures disconnected people from networks of care and support. At its starkest points, these were measures that created distance within healthcare settings, distancing doctors from patients, and families and friends from loved ones in hospital, with significant emotional impact (Dowrick et al., 2021). These impacts stretch beyond frontline healthcare settings, where the sudden inability to see friends and family became a significant issue. Within the museum sector in Northern Ireland, halting provisions such as Alzheimer's support groups sits within this broader context of the impacts of social distancing measures. The emotional stressor of the pandemic was evident in the increasing importance of outreach work during lockdowns and when vulnerable people were shielding. A curator at National Museums Northern Ireland described how their work took on a new significance for participants, one that was far more personal and affecting: 'people were sharing what they were going through in lockdown and if they were struggling a bit or feeling a bit down or not feeling quite themselves or something. It really provided emotional support as well and people were able to share that' (Anon_06). Among those museums that didn't collect objects relating to the pandemic, one of our interviewees reflected that 'none of us had the headspace to go and search out [collections] … we consciously took a step back from that … and looked at ways we could link with people and uplift people' (Anon_02). Here we see a very clear articulation that the museum was to provide a service, in this case through the light-hearted use of social media, to provide a distraction from the challenges associated with the lockdowns.

Concluding thoughts: crisis and the museum

The museum sector is no stranger to continually needing to re-articulate its purpose and relevance, and the challenges posed by the pandemic have extended that need further. In the UK, the pandemic has come after a decade of austerity which has seen cuts to public sector spending in arts and culture (Rex, 2018; 2020). In Northern Ireland, the multiple collapses of the Northern Ireland

Executive and the protracted absence of an Assembly between 2017 and 2020 have led to gaps in governance and leadership in the region (Heenan and Birrell, 2022). During our interviews and focus groups, museum managers repeatedly returned to the concern of 'making sure that we keep the visibility going ... we were very conscious of the importance of keeping our profile going' (Anon_02). In the focus group, a manager of another independent museum told us about the increased need for 'proving your relevance' (FG_Speaker2); a freelancer spoke about 'struggling' with counting value (FG_Speaker1); and museum staff in a Local Authority were described as in a 'whole twist' about how to capture impact when so much about typical delivery was different (FG_Speaker4). All the adaptations demonstrated by museums, and the resilience shown by museum workers gathered by the Museums, Crisis and Covid19 project, are tinged with a need to manage the narrative associated with the museums and the wider creative industries during the pandemic. Evidence that museums adapted to the needs of their audiences is not enough alone; *museums must also be seen to have adapted*. The museum sector is sufficiently self-aware to know that this message needs to be heard by local and central government to enable the sector to continue to build its case for public sector funding.

Robert Janes, editor of *Museum Management and Curatorship*, writes of museums operating in 'perilous times' and reflects on the pandemic as 'a preview and dress rehearsal for the looming climate crisis' (Janes, 2020: 592). As we shift from the global health emergency of recent years to working through the long-term impacts of COVID-19, the sector needs to be alert to how pandemic-related challenges combine with other potential crises facing the museum and heritage sectors. These are revealed by news items and statements coming from the UK Museums Association documenting the impacts of climate change, the cost-of-living crisis, the invasion of Ukraine, disputes around sponsorship, museum closures and debates about anti-racism and decolonisation practices in museums. On the one hand, this suggests a sector facing multiple challenges; on the other, it is a robust sector tackling these challenges directly and collectively.

Despite multiple challenges, the narrative emerging from the museum sector is one of a committed workforce. An interviewee with oversight of the entire Northern Ireland museum sector reflected that 'we have a lot of very passionate, interested and knowledgeable people working in the local museum sector in Northern Ireland, and they have so much to give' (Anon_04). This is akin to what Bakar et al. describe as 'a strong inclination towards work that one loves', or work that 'serves as a vital part of one's self concept' (Bakar et al., 2018: 14–15). The interviewee presents this as a strength of the sector, one that can be combined with support measures to work towards recovery. This shared passion for and commitment to museum work was evident across interviews, focus groups and online discussion forums. Bakar et al. suggest two reasons why people 'work hard': the first is a positive reason – they are passionate about their job and find it engaging; the second reason is negative, with people working hard because of overwhelming work demands and fears around competitiveness and sustainability (Bakar et al., 2018). We suggest the reason why museum staff worked hard through the pandemic lies in both areas. There is no doubt that individuals felt passionate about keeping museums relevant; alongside innovation, there is concern for the lasting impact of the pandemic on the museum landscape – that temporary closures could become long term; that furlough would lead to job losses; and that digital might replace the need for in-person experiences. The dissemination of a narrative of the passionate, committed and agile museum worker is, we suggest, a conscious contribution to efforts to ensure that the value of the sector is continually recognised. While museum staff worked to keep museums relevant during the pandemic, they were also working for the long-term future of the sector.

A curator of a museum in a Local Authority stated that, following the end of social restrictions resulting from the pandemic, 'people [will] want a new emergence, [a] new feeling of doing something they have the right to do' (FG_Speaker4). Although she was referring to museum audiences, the same sentiment was repeated when talking about desire for change within the sector. The disruption brought about by the COVID-19 pandemic will go far beyond a momentary reconfiguration of tasks. The alterations to how we worked, where we worked and the type of work we do have triggered longer-term questions about purpose, intention, the impacts of our practice and what it means personally. Repeated arguments for change, which have come from within the sector and pre-dated the pandemic, have seen more energy and greater traction in the past 2 years (Janes and Sandell, 2019). Feedback from our interviews suggested that the connectivity enabled by online forums organised by museum professionals, advocacy bodies and academic groups has been empowering for museum sector staff in Northern Ireland. The forums enabled new voices and new energy, giving greater pace to the interrogation of museum practice. Hollows (2019) described the activist museum as being a place where the technical and emotional combine. The technical change that was forced by the pandemic enabled the emotion and passion underpinning museum work to come to the fore.

We opened this chapter by citing museum studies scholars and practitioners who have worked for change in the sector. Graham Black suggests that the 'challenge of change' is a 'constant problem for museums, as institutions of continuity and longevity' which are 'comfortable with the status quo' (Black, 2021: 3). The pandemic can be taken as a watershed moment: not only did it disrupt the status quo, it showed that museum staff themselves are what matters most when considering museum value and impact. The versatility demonstrated, and the broader experience gained through how museums adapted, should continue to inform museum practice as attention turns increasingly to issues such as the climate crisis and increases in the cost of living. Seeking to respond to local and global crises and concerns, while adopting an increasingly audience- and community-focused practice, has the potential to bring further challenge and emotional toll on museum workers. One legacy of the pandemic is our demonstration that we can change our practice when it is forced upon us by a crisis; now we must positively lead the change in museums by responding to calls from within and without the sector. This will be integral to ensuring that museums are not simply responding to crises forced upon them, but pre-emptively equipped to support their staff and audiences through these crises as they emerge.

Research respondents

Anon_01 Local Authority Museum Manager. Interview, 8 March 2021

Anon_02 Local Authority Museum Manger. Interview, 12 March 2021

Anon_03 Independent Museum Manager. Interview, 24 March 2021
Anon_04 Advocacy Body Staff Member. Interview, 31 March 2021
Anon_05 Local Authority Museum Manager. Interviews, 4 May and 20 October 2021
Anon_06 Curatorial, National Museums NI. Interview, 7 June 2021
Anon_07 Curatorial, National Museums NI. Interview, 19 October 2021
Anon_08 Visitor Services, National Museums NI. Interview, 18 October 2021
Anon_09 Museum Manager, NI. Interview, 1 March 2021
Brownlee, C. Education Services Officer, Irish Linen Centre & Lisburn Museum [Local Authority museum]. Interview, 20 October 2021
Catney, C. Director of Operations, National Museums NI. Interview, 1 March 2021
Focus Group, five participants: one freelancer, one independent museum manager, two staff from Local Authority museums and one person from the heritage sector. FG1, 10 March and FG2, 28 April 2021
Fryer, M. Outreach Officer, Northern Ireland War Memorial [independent museum]. Interview, 30 April 2021
McGuicken, H. Museum Manager, North Down Museum [Local Authority museum]. Interview, 24 March 2021

Note

1 As part of the Museums, Crisis and Covid19 project, approval was granted from the Ulster University School of Arts and Humanities Research Governance Filter Committee to undertake interviews and hold focus groups with museum staff. Each participant agreed to participate, with some choosing to remain anonymous and others to be named.

References

Agostino, D., Arnaboldi, M. and Lampis, A. (2020), Italian state museums during the COVID-19 crisis: From onsite closure to online openness. *Museum Management and Curatorship*, 35(4), 362–372.
Akkermans, J., Richardson, J. and Kraimer, M. L. (2020), The Covid-19 crisis as career shock: Implications for careers and vocational behaviour. *Journal of Vocational Behavior*, 119, 1–5.

Bajos, N., Jusot, F., Pailhe, A., et al. (2021), When lockdown policies amplify social inequalities in COVID-19 infections: Evidence from a cross-sectional population-based survey in France. *BMC Public Health*, 21(705), 1–10.

Bakar, R. A., Hashim, R. C., Jayasingam, S., et al. (2018), *A Meaningful Life at Work: The Paradox of Wellbeing*. Bingley, UK: Emerald Group Publishing.

Bennett, T. (1995), *The Birth of the Museum: History, Theory, Politics*. London: Routledge.

Black, G. (2021), *Museums and the Challenge of Change: Old Institutions in a New World*. London: Routledge.

Blair, W. (2021), Museums in a time of change/crisis (delete where appropriate). *Museum Ireland*, 27, 21–29.

Blundell, R., Costa Dias, M., Cribb, J., et al. (2022), Inequality and the COVID-19 crisis in the United Kingdom. *Annual Review of Economics*, 14, 607–636.

Bozoğlu, G. (2019), *Museums, Emotion, and Memory Culture: The Politics of the Past in Turkey*. London: Routledge.

Cabinet Office. (2017), *National Risk Register of Civil Emergencies*. London: Cabinet Office.

Christiansen, K. (2020), The Met and the COVID crisis. *Museum Management and Curatorship*, 35(3), 221–224.

Crooke, E. (2021), 'Participation, Trust and Telling Difficult Histories in Museums', in G. Black (ed.), *Museums and the Challenge of Change: Old Institutions in a New World*. London: Routledge, pp. 113–122.

Crooke, E. (2024), 'The Challenge of Change: Museum Practice Informed by and Informing the Peace Process' in L. McAtackney and M. Ó Catháin (eds), *Routledge Handbook of the Northern Ireland Troubles and Peace Process*. London: Routledge, pp. 473–486.

Crooke, E., Farrell-Banks, D., Friel, B., et al. (2022a), *Museums and the Pandemic: Revisiting Purposes and Priorities. A Report of the Museums, Crisis and Covid-19 Project*. Derry/Londonderry: Ulster University.

Crooke, E., Farrell-Banks, D., Friel, B., et al. (2022b), *Museums and Digital Media. A Report of the Museums, Crisis and Covid-19 Project*. Derry/Londonderry: Ulster University.

Crooke, E., Farrell-Banks, D., Friel, B., et al. (2022c), *Museums and Community Wellbeing. A Report of the Museums, Crisis and Covid-19 Project*. Derry/Londonderry: Ulster University.

Deans, P. (2022), 'Crisis Management, Reinvention and Resilience in Museums: The Imperial War Museum during the Second World War Era, 1933–1950' (Unpublished PhD thesis, Newcastle University).

Dickson-Swift, V., James, E. L., Kippen, S., et al. (2009), Researching sensitive topics: Qualitative research as emotion work. *Qualitative Research*, 9(1), 61–79.

Dowrick, A., Mitchinson, L., Hoernke, K., et al. (2021), Re-ordering connections: UK healthcare workers' experiences of emotion

management during the COVID-19 pandemic. *Sociology of Health & Illness*, 43(9), 2156–2177.
Fair Museum Jobs. (2020), A joint statement on the coronavirus pandemic. Available at: https://fairmuseumjobs.org/2020/03/17/a-joint-statement-on-the-coronavirus-pandemic/ (accessed 19 November 2022).
Farrell-Banks, D. (2023), *Affect and Belonging in Political Uses of the Past*. London: Routledge.
Friel, B. and Beavis, J. (2022), The unfolding narrative from Covid-19: Emerging themes and skills in practice. *Eisteach-Irish Journal of Counselling & Psychotherapy*, 22(2), 15–20.
Heenan, D. and Birrell, D. (2022), Exploring responses to the collapse of devolution in Northern Ireland 2017–2020 through the lens of multi-level governance. *Parliamentary Affairs*, 75(3), 596–615.
Hite, L. M. and McDonald, K. S. (2020), Careers after COVID-19: Challenges and changes. *Human Resource Development International*, 23(4), 427–437.
Hochschild, A. R. (1983), *The Managed Heart*. Berkeley, CA: University of California Press.
Hollows, V. (2019), 'The Activist Role of Museum Staff' in R. Janes and R. Sandell (eds), *Museum Activism*. London: Routledge, pp. 91–103.
Irish Linen Centre & Lisburn Museum (ILCLM). (2020), Covid-19 and Me. Available at: www.lisburnmuseum.com/virtual-museum-lisburn/covid-19-and-me-share-your-story/ (accessed 4 July 2022).
Janes, R. and Sandell, R., eds. (2019), *Museum Activism*. London: Routledge.
Janes, R. R. (2020), Museums in perilous times. *Museum Management and Curatorship*, 35(6), 587–598.
Johnston, R., Hogg, R., Martin, G., et al. (2020), *Employment Vulnerabilities in the Arts, Creative, Culture and Heritage Industries as a Result of Covid-19*. Derry/Londonderry: Department for Communities and Ulster University Economic Policy Centre.
Kaplan, F., ed. (1994), *Museums and the Making of 'Ourselves'*. London: Leicester University Press.
Macdonald, S., ed. (2006), *A Companion to Museum Studies*. Oxford: Blackwell Publishing.
Marstine, J. (2011), *Routledge Companion to Museum Ethics*. London: Routledge.
McCreanor, T., Wetherell, M., McConville, A., et al. (2019), New light; friendly soil: Affective–discursive dimensions of Anzac Day commemorations in Aotearoa New Zealand. *Nations and Nationalism*, 25(3), 974–996.
Mellish, T. I., Luzmore, N. J. and Shahbaz, A. A. (2020), Why were the UK and USA unprepared for the COVID-19 pandemic? The systemic weaknesses of neoliberalism: A comparison between the UK, USA, Germany, and South Korea. *Journal of Global Faultlines*, 7(1), 9–45.
Morse, N. (2021), *The Museum as a Space of Social Care*. London: Routledge.

Moura, G. G., Nascimento, C. R. R. and Ferreira, J. M. (2021), COVID-19: Reflections on the crisis, transformation, and interactive processes under development. *Trends in Psychology*, 29, 375–394.

Munro, E. (2014), Doing emotion work in museums; Reconceptualising the role of community engagement practitioners. *Museum and Society*, 12(1), 44–60.

Museums Association. (2022a), Front-of-house charter for change. Available at: www.museumsassociation.org/campaigns/workforce/a-front-of-house-charter-for-change/ (accessed 19 November 2022).

Museums Association. (2022b), Understanding your emotions. Available at: www.museumsassociation.org/careers/wellbeing-hub/understanding-your-emotions/ (accessed 19 November 2022).

National Trust. (2020), We've reduced compulsory job losses following consultation. Available at: www.nationaltrust.org.uk/who-we-are/news/weve-reduced-compulsory-job-losses-following-consultation (accessed 19 November 2022).

Perry, B. L., Aronson, B. and Pescosolido, B. A. (2021), Pandemic precarity: COVID-19 is exposing and exacerbating inequalities in the American heartland. *Proceedings of the National Academy of Sciences*, 118(8), e 2020685118.

Potts, T. (2020), The J. Paul Getty Museum during the coronavirus crisis. *Management and Curatorship*, 35(3), 217–220.

Rex, B. (2018), Exploring relations to documents and documentary infrastructures: The case of museum management after austerity. *Museum and Society*, 16(2), 187–200.

Rex, B. (2020), Which museums to fund? Examining local government decision-making in austerity. *Local Government Studies*, 46(2), 186–205.

Sandahl, J. (2019), The museum definition as the backbone of ICOM. *Museum International*, 71(1–2), 1–9.

Slaughter, J. E., Gabriel, A. S., Ganster, M. L., et al. (2021). Getting worse or getting better? Understanding the antecedents and consequences of emotion profile transitions during COVID-19-induced organizational crisis. *Journal of Applied Psychology*, 106(8), 1118–1136.

Smith, L. (2006), *Uses of Heritage*. London: Routledge.

Smith, L. (2014), Visitor emotion, affect and registers of engagement at museums and heritage sites. *Conservation Science in Cultural Heritage*, 14(2), 125–132.

Smith, L. (2020), *Emotional Heritage: Visitor Engagement at Museums and Heritage Sites*. London: Routledge.

Smith, L., Wetherell, M. and Campbell, G. (2018), *Emotion, Affective Practices, and the Past in the Present*. London: Routledge.

Stanley, B. L., Zanin, A. C., Avalos, B. L., et al. (2021), Collective emotion during collective trauma: A metaphor analysis of the COVID-19 pandemic. *Qualitative Health Research*, 31(10), 1890–1903.

Tolia-Kelly, D., Waterton, E. and Watson, S., eds (2017), *Heritage, Affect and Emotion: Politics, Practices and Infrastructures*. London: Routledge.

Wagner-Pacifici, R. (2021), What is an event and are we in one? *Sociologica*, 15(1), 11–20.

Whitehead, C., Eckersley, S., Daugbjerg, M., et al., eds. (2019), *Dimensions of Heritage and Memory: Multiple Europes and the Politics of Crisis*. London: Routledge.

Witcomb, A. (2015), 'Toward a Pedagogy of Feeling: Understanding How Museums Create a Space for Cross-Cultural Encounters' in A. Witcomb and K. Message (eds), *The International Handbook of Museum Studies: Museum Theory*. Chichester: John Wiley & Sons, pp. 321–344.

Zhou, M. and Kan, M. Y. (2021), The varying impacts of COVID-19 and its related measures in the UK: A year in review. *PloS one*, 16(9), e0257286.

6

Storying older women's immobilities and gender-based violence in the COVID-19 pandemic

Lesley Murray, Amanda Holt and Jessica Moriarty

> During quarantine, my son and daughter-in-law began to neglect my needs. Previously, I did not notice their behaviour, but since all family members must stay home, I started feeling their bad attitude to me. They don't give me food and medicine on time, and they don't even talk to me. Sometimes my daughter-in-law yells at me. I feel like a burden to my family. (Older woman, Kyrgyzstan; Williamson et al., 2021: 28)

In June 2021, the United Nations produced a report on the rise of violence and abuse towards older people during the COVID-19 pandemic. In particular, older people in care homes across the world faced an increased risk of the 'neglect, isolation and lack of adequate services' (UN, 2021: n.p.) that the above quotation describes. The report also highlighted the increase in gender-based violence (GBV) against older people whose mobility was further restricted due to lockdowns (extensive restrictions on movement and measures to promote social distancing that were imposed to control the spread of COVID-19). Here we define GBV as 'a range of "harmful acts" that result from a culture of misogyny, including physical, emotional and sexual violence, rape, stalking and harassment, and are perpetrated over a continuum of mobile spaces' (Murray et al., 2023: 553). The term 'mobile space' refers to the production of space through the movement, or suggestion of movement, of people and things. Studies of GBV during the pandemic (or indeed before the pandemic) do not tend to disaggregate victimisation according to age (Dlamini, 2021). However, evidence suggests that older people can be particularly exposed to GBV perpetrated by their intimate partners, their children and/or their carers, exacerbated as their mobilities are often particularly constrained through societal marginalisation (Murray, 2015). While numerous studies from around the world have found that the more intensified living spaces produced by the lockdowns have led to an increase in GBV (Hourglass, 2020; Peterman et al., 2020), the higher incidence of GBV among older women has not received adequate attention due to the wider invisibility of GBV stories written or spoken by older women.

This chapter draws from a research project that focused on the immobilities of GBV in the COVID-19 pandemic in the UK. Central to this project was the concept of 'immobilities' (Murray and Khan, 2020) to make sense of the range of impacts on physical and imagined movement associated with the pandemic – from the enforced physical restrictions of the COVID-19 lockdowns to the changing sensing of freedom and potential escape, as well as imprisonment, that the intensities of the COVID-19 lockdowns presented. Im/mobilities is a key term in conceptualising the intermittent freedoms and limitations of movement and the control of others' movements – the ways in which movement is privileged. It is particularly relevant in differentiating mobilities, not only according to gender but also to generation (Murray and Robertson, 2016). Conjoining the concepts of generation and mobilities (Murray, 2016) helps us to understand the uneven impacts of the pandemic. COVID-19 is generationed: older people are more likely to feel the impacts of both the disease and the means of controlling the disease by restricting the movements of populations (Age UK, 2021). During the pandemic, people were warned not to visit their older relatives as this would place them at risk. Indeed, in September 2020, the then Secretary of State for Health in England, Matt Hancock, attempted to ensure that young people observed social distancing rules with older people by warning, 'Don't kill your Gran' (*The Times*, 2020: n.p.). In turn, older people were advised to stay at home as much as possible as they were seen to be 'clinically vulnerable' due to their age, regardless of their individual risk (House of Lords Library, 2020).

Importantly for our project, as well as older people being constrained in terms of their own movements and contact with others, the immobilities of the pandemic also made visible injustices that had already existed. The stories that were surfacing during the pandemic told of GBV across lifetimes (Murray et al., 2023). Stories emerged during the pandemic due to the particular conditions in which people were living. Nevertheless, despite the expanse of lives in which older women are more likely to experience GBV, their stories are often obscured in both life-writing and in fiction writing, including works which focus on GBV (Ettorre, 2005). Our research highlights the absence of older women in stories of GBV during the pandemic. We argue that the 'invisibilising' (Priyadarshini et al., 2021) of older women in accounts of GBV not only diminishes our understanding of GBV overall, but creates a new injustice. The chapter thus makes a plea for storytelling as a tool for producing knowledge in research seeking to make visible the lives and experiences of this historically overlooked group.

The invisibilising of older women's experiences of gender-based violence

As Bows (Roberts 2021: n.p.) points out: 'When you look at police data on abuse, rape and murder, older women aren't there. If a crime is looked at, at all, it's treated as a safeguarding issue, gender neutral, "elder abuse" with no perpetrator'. Historically, the ways in which knowledge is produced to make sense of gender-based violence have marginalised older women's experiences. For example, a report by the United Nations Department of Economic and Social Affairs (2013: 1) found that a 'lack of agreed definitions' contributes to the invisibility of older women in domestic abuse evidence. More specifically, older people's experiences of victimisation are excluded from the annual *Crime Survey of England and Wales* (CSEW) as it does not report participants aged 74 years and over[1] and is restricted to participants who live in the community. This is demonstrated in a question put to the House of Lords (2021) by Baroness Gale on 29 July 2020 during an item of business on domestic abuse:

> Question: To ask Her Majesty's Government what plans they have to ensure that any data collected on domestic abuse includes the abuse of people over the age of 74.
>
> Response: My Lords, the Government recognise that the over-74s can be victims of domestic abuse, and we are committed to supporting all victims. The Crime Survey for England and Wales collects data

on victims of domestic abuse, and the most recent assessment of data collection methods did not support raising the age limit for respondents above 74 due to a lower response rate. However, ONS will continue to review the upper age limit. (House of Lords Library, 2021: n.p.)

The omission extends to the important self-completion module on the CSEW, which is designed to ensure victims' privacy when disclosing experiences of domestic abuse, sexual assault and stalking. This exclusion of older people from our national crime survey may contribute to assumptions about older people being at 'low risk' of such violence, when in reality, they are never counted.[2] While police-recorded offences that are flagged as 'domestic-abuse related' do not have the same age-related cut-off, such data are much more susceptible to under-reporting when compared to the CSEW because of victim concerns about stigma, guilt, fear, mistrust and discrimination. Until 2017, the upper age limit for recording of GBV against women was 59 and so there are little historical crime data (Bows, 2019). Nevertheless, recent data indicates that the proportion of violence against the person offences flagged as 'domestic-abuse related' is significant for older women, accounting for 40 per cent of such offences against women aged 75 years and over, and actually *increases* with age for male victims, accounting for 30.3 per cent of such offences against men aged 75 years and over (ONS, 2020). However, most academic research has historically focused on younger people's experiences of GBV (Bows, 2019), with few studies focusing on older people and, in particular, on how gender, class, race and dis/ability intersect with age to produce unique contexts in which gender-based violence can operate.

The little research we do have indicates that older women's experiences of GBV take place within their own unique contours. For example, in their analysis of clients who use MARACs (Multi-Agency Risk Assessment Conferences) to support them through domestic abuse victimisation, SafeLives (Giles, 2016) report that, in cases where the victim is aged 60 years or older, the primary perpetrator is much more likely to be an adult family member (in 44 per cent of cases, compared with 6 per cent of cases involving younger victims); while victims are likely to have experienced a longer period of abuse (6.5 years, compared with 4 years for younger victims) and are much less likely to have attempted to leave the perpetrator (27 per cent of victims over 60 years, compared with 68 per cent of younger victims).

This systematic invisibility in research is mirrored at a conceptual level. Common forms of gender-based violence such as domestic abuse, stalking and harassment tend to be constructed as a 'younger woman's issue', usually falling under the policy directive of 'violence against women and girls'. In contrast, interpersonal violence against older women tends to be conceptualised as 'elder abuse' which, as Holt (2019: 166) has argued elsewhere, 'tends to be framed in the context of institutional care and/or in the context of a care-giving relationship, with the perpetrator in the role of caregiver'. Thus, the gendered and generational contours of GBV against older women tend to be obscured, 'with its characteristics tending to be attributed to the advancing age and associated support needs of the older person, rather than to other dimensions of power that intersect across the life course' (Holt, 2019: 166). This is evident in a recent survey carried out by Hourglass, the safer ageing charity (2020), which found that 30 per cent of respondents did not consider hitting older people as 'abuse', a term that intrinsically acknowledges the role of power within relationships.

Within this context, it is understandable that older women's stories of GBV are missing from women's writing about their own experiences of GBV, whether real or imagined. Their recurrent marginalisation from our national crime survey, in the conceptualisation of GBV and in public understandings of GBV, represents a pre-written story of absence, which can potentially be countered through the self-storying of their own lives by older women.

Storying (older) women's lives

The majority of social groups (and most notably those with intersecting social characteristics) are marginalised in society by the well-established narratives – or pre-written stories – that differentiate them. The pre-writing, in these imagined narratives, of the older female self precludes the storying of their own lives by older women who have experienced, and continue to experience, GBV.

This manifests in various ways, including in how older women are positioned in relation to GBV. Emotionally expressive writing has been studied to investigate its beneficial impact on people's ability to deal with emotional and physical stress (Pennebaker and Beall, 1986). A meta-analysis suggests that writing about emotional topics and life events can lead to significantly improved health outcomes, such as improvements in physical health and wellbeing (Baikie and Wilhelm, 2005). Storytelling can help us make sense of chaotic and confusing events and has often been thought of as central to qualitative research (Gilbert, 2002). Bringing elements of experience, thought and feeling together on one page or text can help researchers identify a central theme or themes that can give clarity to the previously unclear or obscured, and this has obvious benefits for both readers and writers of such texts (Polkinghorne, 1995).

Harvey et al. (1995) identify storytelling as a tool for dealing with loss and trauma among Second World War veterans, evidencing the clear therapeutic benefits. Ellis and Bochner (1992) co-authored a text about their joint decision to have an abortion that helped them to detail and value their individual experience of this shared event, while also using their writing to make connection and better (or differently?) understand what they had been through. Working in this way, storytelling can potentially connect people via shared experiences while also maintaining respect and valuing individual stories and experiences that might not have previously been identified in research. However, despite the life stories that older women may have available to share, there is an absence of such stories, including an absence of autoethnographic accounts. Ettorre (2005) suggests that this is in part related to the ways in which older women's bodies and the older self is more broadly constructed. We acknowledge that asking people to share stories in qualitative research can be difficult at best and retraumatising at worst (Rosenthal, 2003) and that a sensitive, ethical and thoughtful approach to working in this way (as detailed in Parks et al., 2022) is essential.

Plummer (1994) argues that people tell life stories which are not only personal, but which also form part of larger cultural and historical narratives. Narrative puts the personal and the social in the same space, in an overlapping, intricate relationship (Speedy,

2007). Narrative portraiture, building a picture of something through storying, involves working qualitatively with data emerging from interviews, focus groups, observations or other sources that involve people's narratives and can add to the existing field of narrative research by placing the research participants at the centre of the research (Rodríguez-Dorans and Jacobs, 2020). This is highly relevant in relation to experiences with GBV as there are fewer stories about older women – especially autobiographical accounts (Sharratt, 2021). Sharratt points out that Heilbrun's *Writing a Woman's Life* (1989) argues that women's experience is often reduced to normative assumptions of femininity and gendered roles. Looking back at centuries-old stories, she points to *The Book of Margery Kempe* (c. 1436–1438) that tells a story of a mediaeval woman escaping from an abusive marriage by walking the pilgrims' trails. The suggestion is that these associations relating to 'how a woman's life should be' prevail in contemporary narratives (Sharratt, 2021: n.p.). Nevertheless, as will become clear later, it is of paramount importance that we listen out for the stories of older women – particularly around gender-based violence and particularly in the context of the immobilisations of the pandemic.

Storytelling is a method in qualitative research that can address gaps in research in relation to experiences with GBV and seeks to include a diverse range of women, including women aged over 50. Tedlock argues that 'women's ethnographic and autobiographical intentions are often powered by the motive to convince readers of the author's self-worth, to clarify and authenticate their self-images' (Tedlock, 2000: 468). This is, Tedlock argues, a feminist issue. We suggest that storying oneself can offer the necessary detachment that is sometimes needed when seeking a viewpoint from which to examine one's lived experiences, and value this as a meaningful contribution to qualitative research (Moriarty, 2017). This distance can provide a space for reflection that can trigger meaning-making and offer powerful insight into one's own identity. This process can offer women – including older women – a method for authenticating their self-image and recovering feelings of self-worth, allowing for a more expansive sense of self that is able to critique and resist oppressive cultures.

Storytelling in qualitative research, and specifically autoethnography, can provide spaces where the 'weaving of the visual, poetic, and prose narratives is a creative, intuitive, and imaginative process, allowing the body to speak in her own terms' (Metta, 2010: 32). The emphasis on creative stories and lived experiences as research and as a method of valuing research partners means that it offers an appropriate lens through which to view stories of GBV told by women and to value these as equal to traditional academic research. There is some disciplinary divergence here that cannot often be resolved in a transdisciplinary project and so there is a need to sit with the tension. Rather than necessarily analysing these stories, autoethnography in the humanities is more often concerned with valuing the stories and mix of writing styles and acknowledging the individual voices within the research instead (Dundar et al., 2003). Combined with the more analytical autoethnographic approach more common in social science (e.g., Denzin, 2013), we argue that autoethnography is a highly suitable approach for working with and including women of any age who have experienced GBV. Its outcomes can sit alongside more formal analytical approaches or become part of a broader, more formal analytical strategy. The key point here is that storytelling and autoethnography are sources of knowledge that should not be subjugated.

This chapter seeks to encourage conversations in relation to the visibility of older women who have experienced GBV, and to use these conversations to ensure that their experiences are less obscured. We suggest that storytelling, and specifically autoethnography, offers a method of producing research that aspires to needed cultural and social change. We acknowledge the potential tensions within this method, not least between disciplines, and a duty not to reproduce the polarised discourses/ representations that already characterise women's ageing; namely, those that reduce women to frail, unproductive, burdensome and readily-invisibilised bodies, or the 'relentless buoyancy' (Segal, 2013: 179) of privileged bodies, whom Stephen Katz (2005: 188) defines as those who grow old without ageing. Rather, we seek to use stories devised by women over 50 years old to raise awareness and increase understanding, making these bodies and their experiences visible and valued.

Storying the im/mobilities of gender-based violence in COVID-19

In response to the COVID-19 pandemic, the Arts and Humanities Research Council (AHRC) issued a call for transdisciplinary projects offering insights into experiences of lockdown and recommendations for supporting people during this extraordinary time. An aspect of GBV that soon rose to public consciousness during the pandemic was the terrifying rise in domestic abuse, with a 700 per cent increase in helpline calls reported by the UK's largest domestic abuse charity, Refuge. A separate helpline for perpetrators of domestic abuse seeking help to change their behaviour also received 25 per cent more calls after the start of the COVID-19 lockdown (Townsend, 2020). The Immobilities of Gender-Based Violence project was awarded funding by the AHRC and sought to offer people who had experienced GBV dedicated time, a safe and supportive space and methods and techniques to tell their autoethnographic experiences of the pandemic in a variety of ways. The project was structured in several stages. After the initial literature review of existing work in the field, the team devised a new collaborative storying method, 'trans/feminist collaborative autoethnography' (Murray et al., 2022) to include and value the participants as co-authors in disseminated work. We then planned and ran a series of workshops led by writers and artists that would support people who had experienced GBV in lockdown to tell and share stories in a supportive online space. In tandem, we collected 120 existing stories of GBV which were in the public domain. They were gathered from campaign group websites, newspaper reports, magazine stories, policy reports and online blogs. Finally, we analysed the stories collected and made recommendations to inform and change social policies via a series of policy advisor workshops with representatives from the police, health, charities and academia.

We were involved in all aspects of the project, and our research identified that many of the characteristics of the pandemic and its associated lockdowns are risk factors for different forms of GBV – for example, increased stress (and self-medication to manage this), periods of protracted and close proximity with family members and shifts in work and leisure patterns. In particular, many forms of GBV inherently involve 'locking down' – for example, the monitoring involved in coercive control, the surveillance involved in stalking, the lack of passers-by that enables street harassment and sexual assault to go unchecked, and the increased use of digital spaces that enables online forms of abuse to thrive.

We were struck in our research by a number of findings, but three in particular that relate to older women. First is the absence of accounts of older women among the hundreds of stories of GBV in the COVID-19 pandemic in the UK. We analysed these stories ourselves and only two were written by older women. These were both in a report by AGE UK, which focused on critiquing the upper age limit for domestic abuse in crime statistics (as discussed above). Both stories are about experiences of GBV, but not necessarily stories of GBV during the pandemic, which is the second of our findings that relates most perceptibly to older women. Many of the stories that we analysed were not specific to the pandemic, but became visible or *tellable* in the context of the pandemic. As discussed elsewhere (Murray et al., 2023), the pandemic and lockdowns forced a series of resets – including social and cultural. There were changes in the practices of everyday life, as illustrated below by Grace and Sylvia, which meant that women experiencing GBV were subject to a different set of controls and this often allowed them to acknowledge the previous ones – to imagine something different. The changing social, cultural and spatial dynamics of the lockdowns also opened up possibilities for women to physically escape and this in itself then made their stories more tellable.

As the report (Age UK, 2021: 11) says, the stories are 'based on genuine, lived experience – some names and details have been changed to protect the people involved'. The report goes on to say that 'Some of the stories are also an amalgamation of one or more personal stories shared with us by older people'. This is key for us in that it reflected our third suggestion that stories are always a patchwork of recollection, incomplete and partly imagined (Murray et al., 2022). They are always in transition, transforming through the myriad ways in which they are read. Here Age UK became the authors of a new story, one that is the amalgamation of different accounts and echoes their own experience of GBV. The evolution of stories in this way does not detract from their telling of experience. We consider the two stories that we included from Age UK here.

First, Grace who is 81 years old and has endured 57 years of physical and sexual abuse and financial and emotional coercive control by her husband, George.

> I was born in 1938 – the eldest of four children. When father returned from the war he would have rages. We were regularly beaten and made to go to bed without food. It wasn't a happy home.
>
> I put my energy into my studies and started my nurse training. I loved my job and it meant I could leave home.
>
> When I was 22, I met George. He was handsome and charming. He showered me with compliments and made me feel wonderful. We had a small wedding and went on to have three children. Although I enjoyed my job I was thrilled to be at home. I never returned to nursing.
>
> George provided for us financially. However, he controlled every penny and decided what I wore and how I arranged my hair. I lost contact with my friends from work, but he allowed me to chat with the other mothers at the school gates.
>
> George liked routine: evening meal at 5pm, children in bed by 7pm. He had high expectations of what a wife should be and there was no discussion about what I may or may not want.
>
> The only change was on a Thursday. George would go to the races and the children and I would watch *Tops of the Pops*. For years I lived for those Thursdays – laughing and dancing together in the front room.
>
> George would return smelling of whiskey. If he'd won at the races we'd dance, and he'd treat me to a bottle of port. If he'd lost, he'd treat me to a beating. The bruises carefully administered to areas on my body that wouldn't be seen.
>
> When the children left home, George allowed me to have a part-time job. I started to gain confidence and spoke to a friend at work. She helped me realise this wasn't like all marriages, as I'd been told by George. I could stand up to George and say no to his demands.
>
> I began putting money aside for a rainy day. George noticed the change in me and began treating me differently – paying me compliments and taking me out for meals. He even bought me a cat. I adored Misty and she followed me everywhere. I began to believe George had changed and was the man I had met all those years ago.

But one evening, after too much whiskey and a loss at the races, George whispered in my ear what he would do to Misty, if I ever left him. He repeated that threat hundreds of times over the coming years.

His memory has started to fail now. He gets frustrated and angry. Thankfully, problems with his hip mean he can't manage the stairs anymore so he sleeps downstairs and allows me to sleep upstairs.

Night-time is my favourite part of the day. I can rest knowing he can't get to me and feel safe for the first time in years. I lie in bed and my thoughts are completely my own.

And here we are – 57 years of marriage.

'Congratulations, what an achievement!' people say.

If only they knew. (Age UK, 2021: 14)

The importance of this story – and why it needs to be heard – is not just because it voices older women's experience of GBV in the UK, though of course that is important. It is because of the unique vantage point of an older woman's experience of intersecting forms of GBV throughout a lifetime, a story that is likely to have remained unseen and unheard if the pandemic had not created the opportunity. We do not know what this opportunity was, but based on our analysis of other stories, can surmise that, as above, the societal changes associated with the immobilisations of lockdown produced breathing spaces that enabled reflection on past lives (Murray et al., 2023). Also, it may be that the spotlight on GBV presented Age UK with the opportunity to gather stories on GBV, which meant that older women necessarily connected with their past lives. Grace was a young woman when she met George, who would go on to physically assault her for the next six decades. Grace's story tells the tale of the immobilities of GBV, perhaps not during the COVID-19 pandemic, but it is a story that emerged during it. Grace was controlled by George, who dictated how she managed their money and how she dressed and did her hair. She remembers that he was 'charming' and made her feel 'wonderful', an insight into years of gaslighting and coercive control, including not being allowed to work until their children had left home. If all went well for George, he returned from his day out at the races and they danced, a mobile freedom that did not endure. Grace's newfound freedoms in her workplace, both physical and emotional, appear to have provoked George into threatening the life of her pet cat, which she 'adored', as a form of indirect violence or violence by proxy which, as Campbell (2020) has documented, has also increased during the pandemic

It was ultimately *George's* immobility that had brought a significant change to Grace's GBV experience. As he can no longer climb the stairs due to a physical mobility problem, Grace can segregate herself upstairs. She does, however, say that George 'allows' her to sleep upstairs so he still exerts a level of control on her mobility. Her poignant words about night-time being her 'favourite part of the day' suggest that George continues to perpetrate GBV, with the suggestion that he is still controlling her movements and thoughts. Grace's story illustrates the cumulative effects of GBV. It also suggests the usefulness of the concept of generation in framing the intersections of the spatial and temporal in producing GBV. Each generation does not sit in isolation in time and space, but is produced relationally by other generations. We move through from one generation to another, from being part of a younger generation, as Grace was when she first experienced GBV, to an older generation, retaining traces of our generational journey. Grace has absorbed the shared cultures of time and space through the course of her life – she has lived through not only her own experience of GBV, but through the changing socio-cultural constructions of GBV over time. She tells a story of all of those times – from the 1960s to the 2020s. Her own current experience of GBV is determined by her past experiences and how they are remembered and re-remembered. Her new experiences are encumbered with all of these past experiences as we imagine all of our past experiences. And this makes the storying of these life experiences all the more germane. The immobilisations of older women experiencing GBV, which have been illuminated by the COVID-19 pandemic and lockdowns and by their stories, include not only older women being burdened by their lifetime of experiences, but being invisibilised in the present.

The second story from the Age UK report, again told during rather than about the pandemic, is of Sylvia, who is 80, and alongside her husband, Arthur, 'being physically, verbally, financially and emotionally abused' by her adult daughter Paula. They called Age UK's advice line, desperate for help:

> Our daughter was diagnosed with an illness nine years ago which meant she was struggling to cope and had built up lots of debt.

She's our youngest daughter so even though it was difficult for us we wanted to help and care for her. She sold her home to pay off her debts and moved in with us.

We're relieved Paula's health is better now but our lives have become unbearable.

Paula tells us she can't cope with living alone. She's demanded money from us – almost £30,000. She's stopped us seeing our friends and other relatives so we've gradually lost all support and feel so alone.

She shouts terrible things at Arthur and I can see his health deteriorating under the pressure. He has diabetes and breathing problems and all this stress is making him so much worse. I wish I could take it all away for him. (Age UK, 2021: 17)

This story features a very hidden form of GBV, known as child to parent violence. It is only relatively recently that child to parent violence has been recognised as a form of GBV. It made its first policy appearance in the UK Government's action plan *A Call to End Violence against Women and Girls* (HM Government, 2014) and, since that time, has been recognised as an important part of the tapestry in our understandings of how different patterns of domestic abuse emerge across the life course. Yet even within the field of child to parent violence, experiences of *adult* child to parent violence – which is the form most likely to be experienced by older women – are incredibly marginalised. Even in cases of domestic homicide, where age leads to an increased risk in older women, and where older women are as likely to be killed by their sons or grandsons as by their partner, attention in research, policy and practice continues to focus on such violence engaged in by children and adolescents (Bows, 2019; Holt, 2019). The story features a female perpetrator, which is unusual in stories of GBV. Of course, such stories are sparse because most GBV is perpetrated by men (UN Women, 2022). Nevertheless, some women do engage in GBV, often in tandem with male perpetrators and often in cases of so-called honour-based violence, in which violence occurs within a family context in order to 'restore a societal construction of honour' (Gill, 2008: 246). Sylvia's story also illustrates the complexities of gender roles, particularly in terms of caring, with Sylvia placing her husband Arthur as the central character in their shared GBV experience.

Conclusion

Many important research projects developed very quickly in response to the COVID-19 pandemic, but very few of these projects focused specifically on older women's experiences of GBV. Instead, the storying of older women's experiences of GBV was left to organisations such as Age UK and Hourglass. This has meant that older women have, on the whole, been invisibilised, particularly those experiencing intersecting forms of marginalisation, compounded by the isolation of the COVID-19 pandemic and associated lockdowns. We do not know much about Grace and Sylvia's demographic characteristics and whether these have compounded their experience. But we do know that they live in the UK. The first words of this chapter are the story of the older woman from Kyrgyzstan, a country in Central Asia where poverty is high and gender equality is low (World Bank, 2022). Her experience of GBV is both culturally specific and shared across cultures – illustrating the power of storytelling to transcend borders.

Although the stories discussed here do not relate directly to the pandemic, it is the vantage point of the pandemic that is important here. The stories illustrate that GBV does happen to older women and it does happen across lifetimes. We include them here for this reason; they were the only stories about older women in the 120 stories that we analysed during our research. This, in itself, suggests that there is something missing, that older women are being invisibilised from societal accounts of GBV in the same way as they are removed from official crime reporting such as the CSEW. But it is in these rich accounts of lives that we begin to see the temporal as well as spatial patterns of immobilities related to GBV. It is imperative that we find ways to include older women's stories alongside those of other generations.

Moving beyond the lessons of the pandemic, we argue that research which values storytelling should be viewed as equal to conventional academic research. Research that encompasses storytelling, including but not only autoethnography, can address part of the challenge and resistance to dominant and dominating male narratives that are synonymous with traditional academic research. Metta (2016) suggests that telling stories can change dominant and gendered discourses. Working in this way, we hope that, based on the vantage point that the pandemic provided in creating the conditions for more people to tell their stories of GBV, we can create spaces in which older women can articulate their stories beyond it. Appreciating the opportunities of this period of resetting and reflection provides understandings that can be applied to future scenarios, beyond the COVID-19 pandemic.

There is a significant gap in knowledge in our understanding of GBV, the repercussions of which are exacerbated by dominant narratives that are both gendered and generational. Supporting older women to share and tell their stories of GBV can contribute to meaningful societal change around GBV, and this work can be used to inform social policy, improve healthcare services, evolve curriculum design, further democratise research and enhance the lives and experiences of all women who experience GBV. We can then begin to make visible the lives and experiences of older women who experience GBV and reduce any stigma, shame and lack of understanding that have oppressed and invisibilised older women for far too long.

Notes

1 Until 2017, the CSEW excluded participants aged 59 years and over.
2 The most recently available data (ending March 2020) from CSEW suggests that, of people aged 60–74 years, 4.4 per cent of women and 1.9 per cent of men have experienced domestic abuse in the past year (ONS, 2020). The reason that this is the most recently available data is because this module was paused during spring 2020 when the CSEW was moved to a telephone survey because of the lockdown restrictions, thus removing a vital measurement of GBV during COVID-19.

References

Age UK. (2021), *No Age Limit: The Hidden Face of Domestic Abuse*. London: Age UK.
Baikie, K. A. and Wilhelm, K. (2005), Emotional and physical health benefits of expressive writing. *Advances in Psychiatric Treatment*, 11, 338–346. https://doi.org/10.1192/apt.11.5.338
Bows, H. (2019), Domestic homicide of older people (2010–15): A comparative analysis of intimate-partner homicide and parricide cases in the UK.

The British Journal of Social Work, 49(5), 1234–1253. https://doi.org/10.1093/bjsw/bcy108
Bows, H. (2019), *Violence against Older Women, Volume I: Nature and Extent*. Palgrave Studies in Victims and Victimology. London: Palgrave Macmillan.
Campbell, A. M. (2020), An increasing risk of family violence during the Covid-19 pandemic: Strengthening community collaborations to save lives. *Forensic Science International: Reports*, 2. https://doi.org/10.1016/j.fsir.2020.100089
Denzin, N. (2013), *Interpretive Autoethnography*. London: Sage.
Dlamini, N. J. (2021), Gender-based violence, twin pandemic to COVID-19. *Critical Sociology*, 47(4–5), 583–590. https://doi.org/10.1177/0896920520975465
Dundar, C. Jr, Rodriguez, D. and Parker, L. (2003), 'Race, Subjectivity, and the Interview Process' in Jaber F. Gubrium and James Holstein (eds), *Inside Interviewing: New Lenses, New Concerns*. Thousand Oaks, CA: Sage, pp. 11–30.
Ellis, C. and Bochner, A. P. (1992), 'Telling and Performing Personal Stories: The Constraints of Choice in Abortion' in C. Ellis and M. G. Flaherty (eds), *Investigating Subjectivity: Research on Lived Experience*. Thousand Oaks, CA: Sage Publications, pp. 79–101.
Ettorre, E. (2005), Gender, older female bodies and autoethnography: Finding my feminist voice by telling my illness story. *Women's Studies International Forum*, 28(6), 535–546. https://doi.org/10.1016/j.wsif.2005.09.009
Giles, L. (2016), *Older People and Domestic Abuse*. Bristol: SafeLives. Available at: https://safelives.org.uk/sites/default/files/resources/Effective%20support%20for%20older%20people.pdf (accessed 20 September 2022).
Gill, A. (2008), Facts and figures: Ending violence against women. *International Journal of Comparative and Applied Criminal Justice*, 32(2), 243–263.
Harvey, J. H., Stein, S. K. and Scott, P. K. (1995), Fifty years of grief: Accounts and reported psychological reactions of Normandy Invasion veterans. *Journal of Narrative and Life History*, 5(4), 315–332.
HM Government. (2014), *A Call to End Violence against Women and Girls: Action Plan 2014*. London: HM Government.
Holt, A. (2019), 'Violence against Grandparents: Towards a Life Course Approach' in H. Bows (ed.), *Violence against Older Women: Research, Policy and Practice*. Basingstoke: Palgrave Macmillan, pp. 161–180.
Hourglass. (2020). Safer Ageing Press Release. Available at: https://wearehourglass.org/safer-ageing-press-release
House of Lords Library. (2020), Coronavirus, guidance for the over-70s and age discrimination, 3 June. Available at: https://lordslibrary.parliament.uk/coronavirus-guidance-for-the-over-70s-and-age-discrimination/

House of Lords Library. (2021), Domestic abuse of older people, 9 July. Available at: https://lordslibrary.parliament.uk/domestic-abuse-of-older-people/

Gilbert, K. R. (2002), Taking a narrative approach to grief research: Finding meaning in stories. *Death Studies*, 26(3), 223–239. https://doi.org/10.1080/07481180211274

Heilbrun, C. G. (1989), *Writing a Woman's Life*. New York: Ballantine Books.

Katz, S. (2005), *Cultural Aging: Life Course, Lifestyle, and Senior Worlds*. Peterborough, ON: Broadview Press Ltd.

Metta, M. (2010), *Writing Against, Alongside and Beyond Memory: Lifewriting as Reflexive, Poststructuralist Feminist Research Practice*. Bern, Switzerland: Peter Lang.

Metta, M. (2016), 'Embodying Feminist Mothering: Narratives of Resistance through Patriarchal Terrorism from both Mother and Child's Perspectives' in L. Comerford, H. Jackson and K. Kosior (eds), *Feminist Parenting*. Bradford, ON: Demeter Press, pp. 144–167.

Moriarty, J. (2017), 'Writing to Resist: Storying the Self and Audit Culture in Higher Education' in K. Cole and H. Hassel (eds), *Surviving Sexism in Academia: Strategies for Feminist Leadership*. New York: Routledge, pp. 250–258.

Murray, L. (2015), Age-friendly mobilities: A transdisciplinary and intergenerational perspective. *Journal of Transport and Health*, 2(2), 302–307.

Murray, L. (2016), 'Conceptualising Intergenerational Mobilities' in L. Murray and S. Robertson (eds), *Intergenerational Mobilities*. London: Routledge, pp. 1–7.

Murray, L. and Robertson, S., eds (2016), *Intergenerational Mobilities: Relationality, Age and Lifecourse*. London: Routledge.

Murray, L. and Khan, N. (2020), The im/mobilities of 'sometimes' migrating for abortion: Ireland to the UK. *Mobilities* (Special issue), 15(2), 161–172.

Murray, L., Moriarty, J., Holt, A., et al. (2022), Trans/feminist collaborative autoethnographic storying of gender-based violence, during the COVID-19 pandemic. *Journal of Gender-Based Violence* (published online ahead of print). Retrieved Jan 31, 2023, Available at: https://bristoluniversitypressdigital.com/view/journals/jgbv/aop/article-10.1332-239868021X16686970496180/article-10.1332-239868021X16686970496180.xml (accessed 31 January 2023).

Murray, L., Holt, A., Lewis, S., et al. (2023), The unexceptional im/mobilities of gender-based violence in the Covid-19 pandemic. *Mobilities*, 18(3), 552–565. doi: 10.1080/17450101.2022.2118619

Office for National Statistics (ONS). (2020), Domestic Abuse Victim Characteristics, England and Wales: Year Ending March 2020. Available at: www.ons.gov.uk/peoplepopulationandcommunity/crimeandjustice/articles/domesticabusevictimcharacteristicsenglandandwales/yearendingmarch2020#age

Parks, M., Moriarty, J. and Vincent, H. (2022), The immobilities of gender-based violence in lockdown: Devising workshops to support women who experienced gender-based violence during the Covid-19 pandemic to tell and share their stories. *LIRIC: The Lapidus International Research and Innovation Community Journal*, 2(2), 53–75.

Pennebaker, J. W. and Beall, S. K. (1986), Confronting a traumatic event: Toward an understanding of inhibition & disease. *Journal of Abnormal Psychology*, 95, 274–281.

Peterman A., et al. (2020), *Pandemics and Violence against Women and Children*. Working Paper 528, April. Washington, D.C.: Center for Global Development. Available at: www.cgdev.org/publication/pandemics-and-violence-against-women-and-children

Plummer, K. (1994), *Telling Sexual Stories: Power, Change and Social Worlds*. London: Routledge.

Polkinghorne, D. E. (1995), 'Narrative Configuration in Qualitative Analysis' in J. A. Hatch and R. Wisniewski (eds), *Life History and Narrative*. London: The Falmer Press, pp. 5–24.

Priyadarshini, A., Chakraborty, S., Joshi, M., et al. (2021), Women leaders in Bihar invisiblise gender-based violence, blog post. Available at: www.genderandcovid-19.org/research/women-leaders-in-bihar-invisiblise-gender-based-violence/ (accessed 14 September 2022)

Roberts, Y. (2021), End femicide: 278 dead – the hidden scandal of older women killed by men, *The Guardian*, 7 March 2021.

Rodríguez-Dorans, E. and Jacobs, P. (2020), Making narrative portraits: A methodological approach to analysing qualitative data. *International Journal of Social Research Methodology*, 23(6), 611–623.

Rosenthal, G. (2003), The healing effects of storytelling: On the conditions of curative storytelling in the context of research and counseling. *Qualitative Inquiry*, 9(6), 915–933. https://doi.org/10.1177/1077800403254888

Segal, L. (2013), *Out of Time: The Pleasures and Perils of Ageing*. London: Verso.

Sharratt, M. (2021), Life beyond Act One: Why we need more stories about older women, Literary Hub. Available at: https://lithub.com/life-beyond-act-one-why-we-need-more-stories-about-older-women/

Speedy, J. (2007), *Narrative Inquiry and Psychotherapy*. London: Bloomsbury Press.

Tedlock, B. (2000), 'Ethnography and Ethnographic Representation' in N. Denzin and Y. Lincoln (eds), *Handbook of Qualitative Research*. Thousand Oaks, CA: Sage, pp. 455–486.

The Times. (2020), Don't kill Granny with coronavirus says Matt Hancock, 8 September. Available at: www.thetimes.co.uk/article/affluent-youth-are-catching-coronavirus-most-says-matt-hancock-qvbpxw2nk

Townsend, M. (2020), Revealed: Surge in domestic violence during COVID-19 crisis, *Guardian*. Available at: www.theguardian.com/society/2020/apr/12/domestic-violence-surges-seven-hundred-per-cent-uk-coronavirus (accessed 6 September 2022).

United Nations. (2021), Violence against elderly has risen during COVID, UN expert warns, 14 June. Available at: https://news.un.org/en/story/2021/06/1093962

United Nations Department of Economic and Social Affairs. (2013), *Neglect, Abuse and Violence against Older Women*. Available at: www.un.org/esa/socdev/documents/ageing/neglect-abuse-violence-older-women.pdf (accessed 12 September 2022).

UN Women. (2022), Facts and figures: Ending violence against women 2022. Available at: www.unwomen.org/en/what-we-do/ending-violence-against-women/facts-and-figures

Williamson, C., Albone, R., Veitch, G., et al. (2021), *The Impact of COVID-19 on Older People in Low- and Middle-Income Countries: Insights from 2020*. London: HelpAge International.

World Bank. (2022), *Macro Poverty Outlook for Kyrgyz Republic: April 2022 (English)*. Washington, DC: World Bank Group. Available at: http://documents.worldbank.org/curated/en/099007004222229143/IDU038215fde0151a0455909abf0773ada6cc569

7

Empowering obstinate memory: The experiences of Black, Asian and migrant nurses before and during the pandemic

Anandi Ramamurthy and Ken Fero

On 1 April 2020, the news website Al Jazeera published an article titled 'Muslim minority doctors first to die on front line of UK pandemic'. The image accompanying the article revealed that all four doctors were Black (Khan, 2020). Over the previous 2 weeks, other stories of healthcare staff deaths had been reported in the papers; many were Black or Asian, many of them migrant staff. They included Thomas Harvey, a healthcare assistant who had worked for the NHS for 20 years; Mary Agyapong, a young pregnant midwife, who died after giving birth; and John Alagos, a young Filipino nurse of only 23. With no appropriate personal protective equipment (PPE), Thomas Harvey caught COVID-19 in early March 2020. Although his family called the emergency services repeatedly, he was never admitted to hospital (Bartholomew, 2020). He died after collapsing in his own bathroom. Mary Agyapong's family reported that she had felt pressured to work despite being heavily pregnant (BBC, 2020). John Alagos fell ill on his shift, did not have protective equipment to work with COVID-19 positive patients, and had been refused permission to go home when he fell ill (Dickinson, 2020). There were many more stories.

As the rising evidence of the disproportionate impact of coronavirus on Black and Brown communities in the UK became known, explanations began to appear in the press on why we were seeing such disproportionate rates of death. These explanations immediately started to focus on a host of environmental factors: low levels of vitamin D, pre-existing conditions such as diabetes and high blood pressure, cultural factors such as living in extended families and lower socio-economic profiles that lead to poorer housing conditions (Booth and Barr, 2020; Forrest, 2020). While these pre-existing inequalities in health and healthcare were contributory factors to vulnerability, there has been muted discussion of implicit or explicit racialised discriminations in the health sector or more widely in society.

On 19 April 2020, however, an article in the *Nursing Times* suggested that 'BME staff' felt that they were being disproportionately targeted to work on COVID-19 wards (Ford, 2020). Was this contributing to disparities in deaths? As the Equality and Human Rights Commission has highlighted, it is critical to recognise racial discrimination in order to create positive change (EHRC, 2016). Was the feeling that they were being disproportionately targeted to work on COVID-19 wards widespread? If so, why? How did it correlate to previous experiences at work? How have such feelings and experiences created vulnerabilities for both individual staff and the National Health Service (NHS) as a whole? These were some of the questions that the Nursing Narratives: Racism and the Pandemic research project set out to answer through gathering the stories of healthcare workers on film, audio and in text.[1]

While it was clear that doctors were just as impacted as nurses, our decision to focus on nurses, midwives and other healthcare workers was partly made as a result of the early data available on staff deaths, which indicated that the staff group with the greatest number of deaths comprised nursing staff (Cook et al., 2020). In addition, doctors are often more able to have their voices amplified due to their professional position in the health hierarchy. A recent *British Medical Journal* (BMJ) special issue on Racism in Medicine had highlighted the continued inequalities and discriminations faced both by service users and medics in the NHS (Adebowale and Rao, 2020). What, however, was the experience of those whose voices were even more muted?

Our aim was to use storytelling as a methodology to develop our understanding of the impact of historical discriminations on experiences in the COVID-19 pandemic through the experiences of Black, Brown and migrant nurses and midwives. We wanted to recognise their experience and insights as a crucial asset in creating significant change, with which to support the building of a more inclusive society and a more equitable NHS capable of delivering the best patient care. This research was therefore not simply focused on collecting evidence of racial discrimination, but on opening up our understanding of the history of the NHS by placing Black and Brown healthcare workers front and centre in our story of the pandemic. The historical amnesia in the media and wider society on the contribution of Black and Asian people, as well as the muted or silenced representation of the Black and Brown workforce in the NHS during the crisis, have distanced our appreciation of their contribution to the health sector (Simpson et al., 2010). Facts, as Edward Said noted, 'do not at all speak for themselves, but require a socially acceptable narrative to absorb, sustain and circulate them' (Said, 1984: n.p.).

In the Nursing Narratives project, we wanted to explore what role creativity can play in creating the space to not only give suppressed voices 'permission to narrate', but also enable them to be heard. Our outputs aimed to highlight the impact of entrenched and structural racism on a people's approach to a crisis and consider the way forward. Adopting the idea of the 'pandemic as a portal' (Roy, 2020) through which we can reshape our direction as a society, we hoped to create a narrative and shared spaces to deepen societal understanding of the contribution of Black and Brown healthcare workers to our society, celebrate their achievements and create the space for a collective dialogue that could re-envisage the future and take joint action.

Below we outline the theoretical influences and artistic practices that shaped our approach. Critical Race theory offered a framework to understand the experience and impact of racism and highlighted the value of experiential knowledge. Creative methodologies such as A/r/tography's open enquiry, the principles of a 'documentary of force' that emphasise empowerment and political impact for the exposure of 'obstinate memory' and 'third cinema' practices for participation and engagement were methods that influenced our approach.

Critical Race Theory and creative practice

At the root of Critical Race Theory (CRT) is the recognition that 'race' is a social construct and not a biological reality, and that its impact lies not so much in extreme acts of race hatred, but in the everyday experiences of people of colour. CRT scholars argue that because of the way in which racism is embedded in society, a liberal 'colour-blind' approach invariably entrenches racism by its failure to take into account historical injustices and deprivations. If racism is embedded in our thought processes and social structures as deeply as many critics believe, then 'the "ordinary business" of society – the routines, practices, and institutions that we rely on to do the world's work – will keep minorities in subordinate positions'. It is therefore only aggressive, colour-conscious efforts to change the way things are that can challenge the status quo (Delgado and Stefancic, 2017: 27). These challenges may be focused on material and economic demands, as well as on demands to challenge the language and culture of white supremacy. In order to challenge the structures and institutions of power, CRT emphasises the value of experiential knowledge of Black and Brown people. By valuing the subjectivity of experience and centring research in the margins, CRT challenges and resists the suggested objectivity of mainstream research and knowledge (Villenas, 1996).

The focus on experiential knowledge within CRT provides a space to rethink the kind of knowledge considered valuable. The Nursing Narratives: Racism and the Pandemic research project adopted CRT's focus on experience to enable Black and Brown nurses, midwives and other healthcare workers to recount their experiences. Influenced by A/r/tography, which encourages the use of arts practice for qualitative research, we employed a method of open enquiry that is central to allowing expression for empowerment and change (Springgay et al., 2005). Our creative methodology was multi-faceted, using documentary, animation and photography in an attempt to capture under-represented narratives of struggle. Using an arts-based approach which centred emotion as a resource for memory and recovery, our aim was to open up our knowledge and understanding of racialised experiences faced by healthcare workers, through turning our attention towards the unimagined and the uncertain, giving space to the voices and feelings of communities worst affected by the coronavirus pandemic (Greene, 1995).

By enabling Black and Brown nurses to tell their stories through an inclusive, exploratory and expressive methodology, we hoped to gain a better understanding of how the NHS's Workforce Race Equality Standard (WRES) data and the emerging data on the impact of COVID-19 on racialised groups translate into the life experiences of nursing staff, their experience of the pandemic and the people that they care for. We also aimed to increase society's awareness of the contribution of Black British and migrant workers to the NHS. A year into the pandemic, the government's poor understanding of Black and Brown staff experience was highlighted in a House of Commons Public Accounts Committee report on PPE in February 2021. It noted that the government 'does not know enough about the experience of frontline staff, particularly BAME staff' (2021: 8). It asked the government to consider the 'extent to which (and reasons why) BAME staff were less likely to report having access to PPE and more likely to report feeling pressured to work without adequate PPE' (2021: 9). Yet a month later, the *Sewell Report on Race and Ethnic Disparities* denied the existence of structural racism, failing to recognise the impact of racism on health disparities (HMG, 2021). Later in the year, the government's *Coronavirus: Lessons Learned to Date* report (October) recognised that 'the higher incidence' of COVID-19 among racialised communities 'may have resulted from higher exposure to the virus' (HSCC and SCT, 2021: n.p.). However, discussion remained focused on the disproportionate allocation of Black and Brown workers to frontline roles rather than looking more widely at the intersection of interpersonal and structural racisms.

Our grassroots approach to understanding and documenting the experiences of Black and Brown participants from their earliest experiences to the time of writing centred on a participatory process. We met potential participants, answered questions and heard their concerns before engaging in filmed interviews or even framing the interview questions. We used snowballing techniques through existing community networks, as well as a survey and social media, to promote awareness of the project and engage with potential participants who responded to our calls. Trust was a key consideration for participants, and members of the research team's knowledge and participation in the experiences of issues around race and resistance enabled the project and drove its ethos. From the beginning, we knew that we wanted to work in the community and not through NHS Trusts. This, we hoped, would enable participants to speak more freely, as we were aware of the fear of reprisals that many felt. Our aim was not to single out individual Trusts, but draw together stories and patterns of experience to highlight racism within the health service as a national issue that must be addressed. Some members of the team already knew potential participants and had their trust. The filmmaker (Ken Fero) had contacts who were aware of the participatory approach to documentary through previous film productions such as *Ultraviolence* (Fero, 2020). One Co-Investigator was also part of the Caribbean and African Health Network (CAHN) who work to eradicate health inequalities in public health. These personal contacts and the legacy of previous work and commitments around issues of race, justice and representation enabled engagement. They helped participants to have confidence in the research process and the project team.

Despite these avenues of trust, recruitment of participants was not a simple process and many people were wary that the project would just be another piece of research that was carried out without any consequent action. For this reason, we met all those who expressed interest in advance so that they could ask any questions and we could get to know them before filming. Some individuals were very keen, others were afraid to speak out and preferred to take part in audio interviews. This was the case for many Filipino and other migrant nurses. Others decided that although they supported the project, they were not in a position to be interviewed at all. We allowed individuals to make their own decision around the form of participation, unless we were concerned about their vulnerability. This happened in one case, where we advised the individual to carry out an audio interview. There were individuals who, having made the decision to take part, subsequently dropped out of filming on the day. There were also political inconsistencies within one migrant nursing organisation which wanted to take part, gave us significant stories of racism, but then appeared afraid to be involved because we were calling out racism. In the end, of the thirty-seven individuals who expressed a desire to be interviewed on film, twenty attended on the day of filming. They included nurses, midwives and one allied health professional. All these individuals worked, at least in part, for NHS facilities. Two were agency workers at the time of filming. These fluctuating desires to speak or not to speak indicate the tangible fears among health workers about the consequences of speaking out.

Obstinate memory and a documentary of force

In our approach to filming, we adopted the notion of 'obstinate memory' (Fero, 2021). This chronological approach is a filmmaking process that ensures the full capturing of stories over decades. The notion of obstinate memory was employed by Patricio Guzmán to highlight the stories of the disappeared in Pinochet's Chile (Drake, 2015). Over several decades, Guzmán used his documentary practice to expose the brutality of the regime, exploring and exposing the impact of the military junta's use of torture as a form of state control as well as the ongoing national trauma that still exists today. This can be seen, for example, in *Nostalgia for the Light* (Guzmán, 2010). More recently, Fero has employed obstinate memory to document the struggles for justice by the families of Black people killed by police in the UK. Working, for example, with the family of Joy Gardner, a Jamaican student who was killed by the Metropolitan Police in her flat in London in 1993 in front of her 5-year-old son, we follow her mother Myrna as she fights for justice for her daughter. The story is featured in *Justice Denied* (Fero, 1995), *Injustice* (Fero and Mehmood, 2001) and *Burn* (Fero, 2014). Obstinate memory offers an approach where the participants' personal memory (both as individuals and as part of a collective) function as the narrative, thus making interventions that challenge the dominant state narrative (Fero, 2001).

In collecting testimonies, we practised the four elements of a 'documentary of force' – impact, process journalism, approach and formation – a methodology of film practice which focuses on the power and role of film to challenge oppression (Fero, 2018). The desired impact for most conventional documentaries tends to be commercial, educative or entertaining. In a documentary of force, the impact is of a political nature, designed not just to question accepted notions but to directly confront and intervene in the issue. In our film, 'impact' helps to reshape our direction as a society and creates space for participants to offer solutions and re-envisage the future. 'Process journalism' engages with groups of people over an extended period of time in an embedded praxis that challenges what Watkins describes as the 'Monoform', a media form that dominates mainstream television, blurring our understanding and reaction to differing messages to dissipate meaning and our response to human suffering (Watkins, 2004). The participatory process involved in process journalism creates a much more reciprocal power relation between the filmmakers and the participants, borne out by a shared editorial and political direction. 'Approach', one aspect of process journalism, explicitly rejects the 'state of victimology' (Wolfgang, 1957) which holds victims responsible for their own misfortune. Rather than viewing those who may suffer oppression as victims, the emphasis is on the resistance that builds against the cause of that oppression. 'Formation', similarly, emphasises participants developing as organic intellectuals (Gramsci, 1971). Through combining campaigning and the filmmaking process, the aim is to create an environment where participants who may have been victims of oppression are transformed to assume a vanguard position in a struggle.

Documentary of force is a participatory filmmaking process which elicits powerful qualitative data and empowers participants. To reflect this impact, we have included reflections from the participants throughout this chapter:

> I knew that it was a key project and that the stories of lived experience were central to getting the message across to people who disbelieve that racism and privilege are issues that affected the lives of ethnically diverse nurses in the workplace. It was only after filming and when I met a small group of the participants, researchers and sponsors that I fully appreciated the level of collaboration. This was crystallised once I saw the film for the first time at the screening. (Dunn, 2022)

As Felicia reflected:

> Nurses/midwives died during the pandemic and BME nurses/midwives and other healthcare staff were disproportionally impacted at the time. Tackling racism and discrimination is notoriously difficult as it usually means the perpetrators having to/want[ing] to change their heart and minds on how they value BME people. Some of these perpetrators do not want to change or acknowledge the problem. Telling our stories is absolutely powerful in changing the mindsets and is irrefutable as it comes from the person themselves who is describing and relaying their lived experience. (Kwaku, 2022)

The participatory nature of the project created a space where the nurses and midwives involved in the process were able to have input into the narrative content of the film, *Exposed*, that we ultimately produced. Each participant also had editorial control of their testimonies. Conventional documentary production is largely dominated by an expository approach where the narrative is predetermined by a director; however, in this project, we wanted the space and fluidity for experiences, connections and new knowledge to emerge (Nichols, 2001). Following the methodology of a documentary of force, the editorial line in the film was discussed with participants during recruitment, pre-production, the filmed interview and while the project was being edited. We met to discuss the political direction of the film and the key strategies; for example, to debate whether their experience of the segregation of nurses on COVID-19 wards based on race could be described as apartheid.

We documented memory – personal, community, national – as a process of data gathering. This approach facilitated a reflective memory, one that is able to speak of the past, show the present and question the future. This reflexive process was carried out by the film participants who were able to do so in a forensic manner as they were given unlimited space and time to do so:

> I did not know what to expect and the approach to capturing my story was unhurried, allowing it to unfold and flow. I did journey back to situations that forced me to think about certain individuals and attitudes that caused me concern. These were few in number and did not deter me. I did reflect on how I stood up to some of this, and get over or through any obstacles that were put in my way and manage to achieve the career progression that I sought. (Dunn, 2022)

The approach to the interviews was to ensure that a space was created where participants could feel at ease and also in control of the situation. One of the major concerns that informed the filming was the awareness that many of the participants would be recalling very traumatic experiences, and an approach was needed that could ensure a safe environment where the emotions that emerged were therapeutic and not exploitative. We provided space and time for participants with no limits to the amount of filming and no restrictions on what could be said.

The element of 'process journalism' provides the critical time for engagement, reflection and adjustment. This is part of the 'formation' aspect of a documentary of force outlined earlier; it included individual and group interactions online and in person. While this was very effective in practice, we did have several meetings with potential participants who declined to take part; in many cases, the fear of reprisals or victimisation if they had gone public by appearing in the film was a risk they could not take. For those who committed to the project, we had conversations about possible workplace reprisals and how they would be dealt with and what support we could give. In terms of the process, they were briefed in advance and were informed that the interviewing technique was conversational and not inquisitorial. There was no need for them to 'prepare', alleviating any pressure on them to memorise factual evidence.

> I felt safe and supported and there was no judgement, or censoring of my lived experience. I felt very emotional at times reliving some of my experiences, but I also felt safe to tell the truth, I felt empowered as well, like this could make a difference and maybe, me telling my story will encourage others to in the future. (Newbold, 2022)

Despite the possibilities of retribution from employers given the historical 'silencing' of the voices of Black, Asian and migrant nurses, participants' decisions to take part in the project were driven by bravery and the desire to challenge authority:

> I took part in the project to try and make a change to the systemic racism in the NHS, to be able to share my story safely, without judgement or gaslighting, I also took part to make some good from the racism I've experienced my whole nursing career and continue to face, in the hope that the film will raise awareness and prevent more nurses of colour experiencing what I did. (Newbold, 2022)

The process was an emotional journey for many of the participants, highlighting courage and raising questions and concerns:

> It was very emotional reliving the experiences. I was upset at some points and had mixed feelings: '[I]s it going to be the same outcome as with other projects on the subject?' After the interview there were more mixed feelings about when the film is being showed all over the place and my [T]rust management sees it. What will it mean for me, employment wise? I didn't really want to care much about the job though, I have that feeling that I am doing the right thing, by participating to help others in the future, who might not have as much

> courage and cause themselves harm. Having the manifesto of change already in place may prevent this. (Babalola, 2022)

Obstinate memory allows participants to make a more reflexive response to research questions, enabling the emergence of patterns. With memories of decades of experiencing wrongdoing, they are able to process, analyse and, most importantly, offer a critique for resistance. Viewing participants not as victims, but as experts, enabled them to present their story as well as comment on medical, social and political aspects of the story, from a personal and informed point of view. The testimonies provide important evidence for the continued issue of accountability, while deepening societal understanding of the critical contribution of Black, Asian and migrant nurses and midwives during the pandemic. While recognising their experience of victimisation, they also develop critical commentary contributing to current debates on anti-racism in the health service, which was empowering and was recognised by participants as such.

> It actually took me a while to watch my own testimony, when I did decide to watch it, I was anxious as to what I had said. After watching my own and others' testimonies, I felt that I was not alone and that doing this film was so needed and important for the public and wider audiences to hear our stories and understand how and why so many of our BAME staff had died. They needed to hear the truth and facts. (Anwar, 2022)

The extended interviews from a filmmaking process influenced by the concept of obstinate memory created an archive that can be a valuable resource for reflection for the profession as well as for further academic research. While the collective documentary highlighted key themes that we encountered in the experience of nurses, we were aware that this does not enable an understanding of the relentless nature of racism that an individual can experience; nor does it enable an understanding of the compounding impact of racialised trauma. We therefore decided to produce, with consent from the participants, a series of individual full-length testimonies which are housed in a digital online repository (https://nursingnarratives.com/film-testimonies/). This was a core output of the project in terms of preserving stories for future generations. Collectively, the testimonies highlight the importance of recognising the differential impact of COVID-19 on communities in any memorialisation.

The emphasis on challenging victimology and viewing the participants as organic intellectuals in their struggle for justice led to the creation of an 'Anti-Racist Manifesto for the Health Service'. The manifesto reflects the major concerns of the participants made apparent through the filmmaking process. Through an iterative process, it was agreed by both the film and audio participants. Once the interviews were recorded and transcribed, clear themes and shared experiences emerged that pointed to critical issues that the participants outlined individually. For some in their senior roles, it became clear through a series of online group meetings that a collective response to these points might help to galvanise a collective response from nurses and midwives across the UK. We suggested it could take the form of a manifesto. All participants were involved in the writing and editing of the document in conjunction with the research team. It is worth reading and reflecting on in full as it is an important collective effort by Black, Asian and migrant healthcare workers to present demands based on their own experience at this critical time in the NHS.

An Anti-Racist Health Service – A Manifesto for Change

Due to the history of racist practices towards Black and Brown health workers that have been further exposed by our experience of the pandemic, we demand a health service that is actively anti-racist:

We call upon the NHS to:

1. Implement a Zero tolerance to racism policy and practice.
2. Stop putting Black and Brown staff in danger of death and psychological harm.
3. Build a more compassionate NHS with respect and equity for Black and Brown workers.
4. Remove whiteness as the benchmark in training and organisational culture.
5. Build an NHS with equality at the core of health provision for all ethnicities.
6. Create clear and real consequences for racist actions, including dismissal, legal action and referral to regulatory bodies.
7. Create a fair and transparent recruitment process, including all internal opportunities.
8. End the exploitation of Black and Brown workers – delegate work equitably.

We call upon Universities and Practice learning partners to:

9. Be accountable for providing equitable access to learning opportunities that enable all student nurses and midwives to meet the Nursing and Midwifery Council (NMC) competencies for registration.

We call upon the government and regulators to:

10. Create accountability and penalties for trusts for failure to address racism through the Health and Safety Executive.
11. Recognise the experience and training of overseas nurses and midwives. Don't treat them automatically as unqualified.
12. Evaluate and reflect on Black and Brown staff experiences of discrimination in Care Quality Commission (CQC) ratings.
13. Investigate and challenge referrals of Black and Brown nurses and midwives to regulatory bodies with no evidence and no case to answer.
14. Change the immigration system for international healthcare workers to end exploitative visa fees, the denial of recourse to public funds and give automatic indefinite leave to remain.
15. Reinstate third party discrimination into legislation.

We call on all Black and Brown staff to build a collective voice, which will also be supported by all allies to build a just health service.

The manifesto is housed on the Nursing Narratives website. It is being used as a campaigning tool, with nurses' and midwifery organisations disseminating it widely. The manifesto has also been taken up as a template by Black and Brown nurses internationally, to encourage reflections on their own circumstances. For example, at a recent film festival in Malmö where the film was screened, the project participants built campaigning links with nurses from Sweden and Norway who are keen to adapt the manifesto to their own particular circumstances.

Opening up the narrative space

Exposed, the documentary film that we ultimately produced, was presented as a collaborative voice, one where participant testimonies intersected in a mosaic to create a collective narrative. The story segments selected in the documentary were influenced by the content of both the filmed and audio interviews. The interweaving of individual stories in a consultative editing process aimed to present a national picture. We were conscious of the difficulties that we had had in recruiting migrant nurses to the project. The precarious immigration status of some participants placed migrant nurses in a particularly vulnerable position, since a disciplinary action at work or loss of employment could end in deportation – a racialised and brutal state strategy. Their personal responsibilities, often as the main source of income for their families abroad, was an additional pressure. We therefore ended up with very few migrant nurse participants who were able to be filmed. This inevitably muted their visual representation. Out of the two migrant nurses who did come forward for the film, we anonymised one migrant nurse participant to protect them. The other was clear that she wanted to speak out publicly.

In the production of *Exposed* (Fero and Ramamurthy, 2022), we were influenced by the filming practice of third cinema, a film movement that grew out of liberation theology and adopted film as a political practice made in conjunction with the people, to reflect their lived reality and their political critiques (Getino and Solanas, 1971). For third cinema practitioners, 'the capacity for synthesis and the penetration of the film image, the possibilities offered by the living document, and naked reality, and the power of enlightenment of audio-visual means make the film far more effective than any other tool of communication' (Getino and Solanas, 1971: 122). Documentary, in particular, offered a form that could be the basis of revolutionary filmmaking:

> Every image that documents, bears witness to, refutes or deepens the truth of a situation is something more than a film image or purely artistic fact; it becomes something which the System finds indigestible. Testimony about a national reality is also an inestimable means of dialogue and knowledge on the world plane. (Getino and Solanas, 1971: 123–124)

By intercutting the stories of nineteen participants we created a tapestry of their experience that spoke truth to power. The collective narrative was edited to reflect the narratives of those who could not speak in the film but contributed to the research. The findings of the overall project included the results of a survey with

308 respondents, and narrative interviews with 45 individuals. Despite the difficulty in capturing the experience of many migrant nurses from the global south on film due to their vulnerability, we were able to use our wider knowledge from the audio interviews to ensure that key experiences of vulnerability and exploitation for migrant nurses were highlighted.

To challenge racism, *Exposed* not only recounted stories of racism faced by Black and Brown staff in the pandemic and in their working lives, but centred Black and Brown healthcare staff within the frame. The film gives space to their experience of the unfolding pandemic and the trauma that healthcare staff experienced. Roseline describes hiding from her son to keep him safe and lying to him about the devastating experience of losing six patients in one day to protect him from trauma. Others speak of the UK's lack of preparedness: 'We were all scared, we were all lost.' Through these reflections, the role of Black and Brown health workers is afforded value and dignity.

The overall findings of the project highlighted key issues that impacted on the experience of Black and Brown nurses and midwives in the pandemic. These include a widespread culture of racism that permeates daily practice, with racialised stereotypes and attitudes accepted as the norm. This culture has led to the exclusion and neglect of Black and Brown staff; many described being 'pushed out', made 'invisible' and side-lined from critical discussions. It is a culture that routinely leads to Black and Brown health workers being given heavier and more risky work. It is a culture that leads to Black and Brown health workers being constantly overlooked for progression.

During the pandemic, such practices meant that Black and Brown staff were often the first to be put in situations of risk, with poor attention to their welfare, lack of PPE and risk assessments described as a tick box exercise:

> Was it because we're undervalued that they didn't step up to ensure that we were protected? Because that's what it feels like. (Anwar, 2022)

> Staff were threatened with their work permits to be revoked during that time as well, several of the staff said they couldn't challenge the decision because if they did they would be faced with bullying and harassment at work. (Kwaku, 2022)

Agency workers described how they first thought they were not being given PPE because they were agency workers, but then they realised that many of their Black and Brown colleagues were being treated similarly: 'I was allocated to a COVID ward and I was not given protection, I asked for like a proper filtered mask and I was told I can't have it because I will scare people' (Bennett, 2022).

Some described what can be seen as a cultural apartheid: 'In the Emergency Area they divided into different sections, the red area and the green area. All the Black nurses were always allocated in the red area which was more dangerous' (Ajose, 2022).

In order to reflect on the collective experiences above and because we were limited to filming in a controlled studio during the pandemic, we created animations to thread each section of the film together. We aimed to create moments of pause and reflection to increase the power of the narrated experiences. The visuals and voiceover create a series of provocations. Some elicit the feeling of forensic medical investigations through the blue/black colours of X-rays held up to the light. Often tampered with or damaged, these images call on the viewer to look deeper, beyond the surface. In one, the sign 'Blacks Only' flashing on a TV screen recalls the exclusionary signs of the colour bar; this time, the sign ironically turns the former exclusion around to include only Blacks in the space of danger.

The animated sections allow the viewer to reflect on wider political strategies of corporations and governments in relation to death and crisis and on the historical experiences of racism and migration. Evoking philosophical and political thinkers such as Naomi Klein and Frantz Fanon, we aimed to encourage the viewer to reconsider dominant media narratives of the pandemic and give greater weight and authority to the voices of Black and Brown health workers in the film. The narrator questions the feeling of a wartime spirit and a nation 'in it together', suggesting that the state's pandemic response was part of 'the shock doctrine' (Klein, 2007) that evokes fear and panic as a means of social control. As we move through the story, the narrator alludes to Frantz Fanon's critique of racism to highlight both an entrenched colonial past and the psychological impact of racialisation (Fanon, 1967). The authoritative, restrained voice acts as a contrast to the emotional narratives and reflections of the health workers, enabling their speech to be heard with a stronger force.

As we move through the film, the health workers' reflections expand to include not just their own experience, but their response to the death of George Floyd (May 2020) and the Black Lives Matter movement (BLM), recognising their role as organic intellectuals: 'It was like opening a wound that was still bleeding' (Fatimah Ghaouch, 2020 interview). The 2020 BLM protests were a significant moment that enabled many nurses and midwives to get organised. As a third cinema practice, highlighting 'the ways of organising and arming for the change' was crucial (Getino and Solanas, 1971: 125). Neomi reflects on the significance of Black Lives Matter:

> Black and Brown nurses need their own organisation so that they can be allowed a voice together. Black Lives Matter inspired me so much. I felt this is a platform and an opportunity for me to speak out about the injustices that I have experienced from the day I was born in this country because we were suffering in silence. (Bennett, 2022)

Both the principles of third cinema and a 'documentary of force' use film to catalyse progressive or revolutionary change. Our aim was to create impact at many levels. While the film was released online for general viewing supported by a press and social media campaign, one of the important intentions was to hold screenings with Q&As with the participants to create a space for the narrative to be extended through discussion with other nurses. At every screening, Black and Brown healthcareworkers, young and old, who have come to watch the film, have spoken out about their own experiences of racism. White allies have expressed shock and a sense of shame. These experiences have been most powerfully felt at our in-person screenings, where emotions gain a physical presence and resonance that cannot be achieved in an online meeting. The London premiere of the film in July 2022 was such an event:

> People are always very emotional. At the last screening in London, several people in the audience had also experienced race discrimination. So often in the question and answer sessions for the panel, this turns into the audience relaying their trauma and for some of them, this is a cry for help. (Kwaku, 2022)

The film continues to be screened around the UK. Our aim is for participants and audiences to debate, contribute and organise:

> I have found audiences to be shocked and emotional when listening to and viewing the content. It invariably led to people committing to action to change. Invariably, people spent time wanting to talk about what they could do and increasingly, how they may do it with others in partnership across a system. That said, we need more people to view the film and, in particular, those who do not see racism as an issue in their workplace or community. Worse still, those who are aware of it and either turn a blind eye or participate in it. These are the mindsets that need to change, these are the people who need to experience dissonance in order to dismantle their current views around race and justice. (Dunn, 2022)

We continue to try to ensure that one or two participants take part in the Q&As at other screenings as much as possible, to create a discursive space that allows for embellishment, awareness and progress. But this needs sustained work:

> The experience of the screenings and people's reactions to the film ha[ve] been diverse, there are some spontaneous reactions by people who have started to act forming network groups including allies to drive this forward. Some reactions of surprise, soul searching and reality during the discussion at the screening which sometimes they want to divert to previous things or documents in place about equality, discrimination and bullying. However, it takes great effort to keep the screenings focused on the film and the manifesto for change including what is expected of the organisation. (Dunn, 2022)

Speaking 'truth to power' was one of our aims and there have been some positive responses. Paul Roberts, the Chief Executive of Gloucestershire Health and Care NHS Foundation Trust, made the following response (by email to Ken Fero) following the screening of *Exposed* and Q&A on 20 July 2022:

> In the discussion after the film screening, we heard from nurses locally who spoke about how they have spent 30 years trying to change racist attitudes that still persist today, causing untold harm, distress and getting in the way of career satisfaction and progression. We can't allow this to happen in our Trust. It's about actively changing and challenging and it's not up to the colleagues among us who are from minority ethnic groups to bring about the change – it's all of us. (Roberts 2022)

One of the earliest screenings of the film was held at the Royal College of Nursing Congress 2022. Subsequently, many regional officers began to take up the opportunity of screenings across the country. Ali Upton, Chair of the Royal College of Nursing UK Health & Safety Representatives Committee, made the following comment (by email to Ken Fero) following a viewing of *Exposed*:

> The sadness behind *Exposed* is that the racism, bullying and harassment these 19 colleagues have openly talked about is only a small account of the toxicity that exists in healthcare. We must collectively work together to ensure that this behaviour does not continue, and employers have a zero tolerance. A quote from the film that stays with me and shows the direction we must all take: 'Not everything that is faced can be changed, but nothing can be changed until it is faced'.

The film *Exposed* has not only been employed to bring about change and give voice to those whose narratives have been silenced, but has acted to empower the individuals who took part to develop as organic intellectuals in their communities. Many of the participants have spoken about the positive experience of taking part:

> It has really had a positive impact on my confidence and drive to keep raising awareness and fighting for action to fight racism and hold perpetrators accountable for their racist behaviours. (Newbold, 2022)

> This experience of being involved in the project has impacted me personally moving forward in my career and politically pushing this through the [T]rust, union and my MP. (Babalola, 2022)

> I am standing with every person who contributed to the making of this film. I would be there in a heartbeat if any of the participants needed support for an issue or event. I feel that we have shared something profound and share a connection. (Dunn, 2022)

By using obstinate memory within a documentary of force we were able to consolidate ideas for collective struggle, sown through interactions during research, interviewing, editing and screenings. These were sites of political conversations and alignments as much as they were about the process of academic research and cultural production. The idea for the Anti-Racist Manifesto for the Health Service and the subsequent solidarity actions which the filmmaking process helped to consolidate build on the personal and community histories of the Black and Brown nurses and midwives. At the same time, the political activism in other struggles around race and resistance by the project team created a spirit of subjectivity (being influenced by people's feelings and thoughts) that is essential to move beyond data collection. As Jean-Luc Godard argued, 'The problem is not to make political films, but to make films politically' (Godard, 1970, quoted in Hoberman, 2005: para. 1). This is exactly what a methodology of a documentary of force can deliver.

In conclusion, it is only right in a project of this nature to give the last word to one of the participants, speaking in *Exposed* to the struggle against racism: 'Black and [B]rown nurses need their own organisation so that collectively they can be a loud voice together. There are common themes across the country, at the moment they are fragmented but we're all saying the same thing, our experiences are mirror images of each other' (Bennett, 2022).

Research project participants

Ajose, Roseline (2022), Nursing Narratives Participant Post-project Participant Survey

Anwar, Nafiza (2022), Nursing Narratives Participant Post-project Participant Survey

Babalola, Olanike (2022), Nursing Narratives Participant Post-project Participant Survey

Bennett, Neomi (2022), Nursing Narratives Participant Post-project Participant Survey

Dunn, Estephanie (2022), Nursing Narratives Participant Post-project Participant Survey

Kwaku, Felicia (2022), Nursing Narratives Participant Post-project Participant Survey

Newbold, Gemma (2022), Nursing Narratives Participant Post-project Participant Survey

Note

1 Ethics review for the Nursing Narratives: Racism and the Pandemic Research Project was carried out by Sheffield Hallam University ethics review committee. Ethics Review no: ER26917892.

References

Adebowale, V. and Rao, M., eds (2020), Racism in medicine. *British Medical Journal* (special issue, February). Available at: www.bmj.com/racism-in-medicine

Bartholomew, E. (2020), 'Devoted' father-of-seven NHS worker from Hackney 'died alone of coronavirus after treating infected patient', *Hackney Gazette*, 31 March. Available at: www.hackneygazette.co.uk/news/22931804.devoted-father-of-seven-nhs-worker-hackney-died-alone-coronavirus-treating-infected-patient/

BBC. (2020), A pregnant nurse who died with Covid-19 felt 'pressurised' to go to work, 23 March. Available at: www.bbc.co.uk/news/uk-england-beds-bucks-herts-5649897

Booth, R. and Barr, C. (2020), Black people four times more likely to die from Covid-19, 7 May. Available at: www.theguardian.com/world/2020/may/07/black-people-four-times-more-likely-to-die-from-covid-19-ons-finds

Cook, T., Kursumovic, E. and Lennane, S. (2020), Exclusive: Deaths of NHS staff from covid-19 analysed. *Health Service Journal*, 22 April. Available at: www.hsj.co.uk/exclusive-deaths-of-nhs-staff-from-covid-19-analysed/7027471.article

Delgado, R. and Stefancic, J. (2017), *Critical Race Theory: An Introduction* (3rd edition). New York: New York University Press. https://doi.org/10.18574/9781479851393

Dickinson, E. (2020), Nurse, 23, dies after 12-hour shift treating Covid-19 patients 'without adequate PPE', Chronicle Live, 5 April. Available at: www.chroniclelive.co.uk/news/uk-news/nurse-23-dies-after-12-18046632

Drake, Chris (2015), Desert of the disappeared: Patricio Guzmán on Nostalgia for the Light, BFI, 19 February. Available at: www.bfi.org.uk/news-opinion/sightsound-magazine/interviews/desert-disappeared-patricio-guzman-nostalgia-light

EHRC. (2016), *Healing a Divided Britain: The Need for a Comprehensive Race Equality Strategy*. Equalities and Human Rights Commission. Available at: www.equalityhumanrights.com/sites/default/files/healing_a_divided_britain_-_the_need_for_a_comprehensive_race_equality_strategy_final.pdf

Fanon, Frantz (1967), *Black Skins, White Masks*. Paris: Éditions du Seuil.

Fero, K. (1995), *Justice Denied* (film). London: Migrant Media.

Fero, K. (2014), *Burn* (film). London: Migrant Media.

Fero, K. (2018), 'Documentary Practice as Radical Process in Challenging Dominant Media and State Narratives' (unpublished PhD thesis, Sheffield Hallam University). Available at: http://shura.shu.ac.uk/23304/1/Fero_2018_PhD_ChallengingDominantMedia.pdf

Fero, K. (2020), *Ultraviolence* (film). London: Migrant Media.

Fero, K. (2021), Obstinate memory: Documentary as trauma in disrupting state narratives on racial violence. *Viewfinder Magazine*. Available at: https://learningonscreen.ac.uk/viewfinder/articles/obstinate-memory-documentary-as-trauma-in-disrupting-state-narratives-on-racial-violence/

Fero, K. and Mehmood, T. (2001), *Injustice* (film, 98 minutes). London: Migrant Media. Available at: https://vimeo.com/34633260

Fero, K. and Ramamurthy, A. (2022), *Exposed* (film). Sheffield: Sheffield Hallam University.

Ford, Megan (2020), BME nurses 'feel targeted' to work on Covid-19 wards, 19 April . Available at: www.nursingtimes.net/news/coronavirus/exclusive-bme-nurses-feel-targeted-to-work-on-covid-19-wards-17-04-2020/

Forrest, Adam (2020), Black men suffer highest coronavirus death rate in UK, government figures show, *Independent*, 19 June. Available at: www.independent.co.uk/news/health/coronavirus-deaths-uk-black-men-ethnicity-ons-a9574796.html?r=85458

Getino, Octavio and Solanas, Fernando (1971), Towards a third cinema. *Tricontinental*, 14 (October), 107–132. Havana: Organización de Solidaridad de los Pueblos de África, Asia y América Latina. Available at: https://ufsinfronteradotcom.files.wordpress.com/2011/05/tercer-cine-getino-solonas-19691.pdf (accessed 1 September 2022).

Godard, Jean-Luc (1970), *What Is to Be Done? Manifesto of the Dziga Vertov Group*. London: After Image.

Gramsci, A. (1971). *Prison Notebooks*. London: Lawrence & Wishart.

Greene, M. (1995), *Releasing the Imagination: Essays on Education, the Arts, and Social Change*. San Francisco, CA: Jossey-Bass (Wiley).

Guzmán, P. (2010), *Nostalgia for the Light* (film). New York: Icarus Films.

HMG. (2021), *Commission on Race and Ethnic Disparities: The Report*. London: Her Majesty's Government.

Hoberman, J. (2005), *Tout va bien* revisited, The Criterion Collection, 14 February. Available at: www.criterion.com/current/posts/356-tout-va-bien-revisited

House of Commons Public Accounts Committee. (2021), *COVID-19: Government Procurement and Supply of Personal Protective Equipment*. Available at: https://committees.parliament.uk/publications/4607/documents/46709/default/

HSCC and STC. (2021), *Coronavirus: Lessons Learned to Date*. Health and Social Care Committee and Science and Technology Committee, UK Parliament, 12 October. Available at: https://committees.parliament.uk/committee/81/health-and-social-care-committee/news/157991/coronavirus-lessons-learned-to-date-report-published/

Khan, Aina (2020). Muslim minority doctors first to die on frontline of UK pandemic, *Al Jazeera*, 1 April. Available at:www.aljazeera.com/news/2020/4/1/muslim-minority-doctors-first-to-die-on-front-line-of-uk-pandemic

Klein, Naomi (2007), *The Shock Doctrine: The Rise Of Disaster Capitalism*. Toronto, ON: Knopf.

Nichols, B. (2001), *Introduction to Documentary*. Indiana: Indiana University Press.
Roy, Arundhati (2020), The pandemic is a portal, *Financial Times*, 3 April.
Said, Edward (1984), Permission to narrate. *Journal of Palestine Studies*, 13(3), 27–48. doi: 10.2307/2536688
Simpson, J. M., Esmail, A., Kalra, V.S., et al. (2010), Writing migrants back into NHS history: Addressing a 'collective amnesia' and its policy implications. *Journal of the Royal Society of Medicine*, 103(10), 392–396. doi: 10.1258/jrsm.2010.100222
Springgay, S., Irwin, R. L. and Kind, S. W. (2005), A/r/tography as living inquiry through art and text. *Qualitative Inquiry*, 11(6), 897–912.
Villenas, S. (1996), The colonizer/colonized Chicana ethnographer: Identity, marginalization, and co-optation in the field. *Harvard Educational Review*, 66(4), 711–731. https://doi.org/10.17763/haer.66.4.3483672630865482
Watkins, Peter (2004), The global media crisis. Available at: http://pwatkins.mnsi.net/dsom.htm (accessed 1 September 2022).
Wolfgang, Martin F. (1957), Victim precipitated criminal homicide. *Journal of Criminal Law and Criminology*, 48(1), 1–11.

8

The shameful dead: Vaccine hesitancy, shame and necropolitics during COVID-19

Fred Cooper, Luna Dolezal and Arthur Rose

On 24 August 2021, the online media platform New Frame published a satirical cartoon by the South African illustrator Carlos Amato. The cartoon depicts several rows of gravestones, each etched with a trope from vaccine-hesitant discourses: 'My body my choice', 'I trust my own immune system', 'Who stands to gain?', 'They developed it too fast', 'Free thinker', 'Did my own research' (Amato, 2021). Whether through circulation of Amato's cartoon or a like-minded perspective on the situation, photographs of homemade Halloween decorations with identical imagery were widely shared on social media later that year (Kronbauer, 2021). This trope – in which the poor judgement of the unvaccinated coronavirus (COVID-19) dead stands as their epitaph – crystallised a nexus of social and political shaming around vaccine hesitancy or refusal in countries with mass vaccination programmes. Frequently, shame has been directed at individuals posthumously; for example, in the online sharing of obituaries for notable or vocal anti-vaxxers (Levin, 2021). While some of the most visible instances of 'death shaming' have been decried, they nonetheless remain as extreme iterations – and a logical product – of a more pervasive culture of shame over vaccination, or lack of it. Rather than paying close attention to the contexts (including a trusting and shame-less engagement with public health messaging and communication) which enable different publics to make informed decisions about vaccination, the 'unvaccinated' have increasingly taken on the characteristics of a shamed population, culpable for the spread of the virus, for other adverse health outcomes produced by a health system under strain, for the threat of future public health restrictions to everyday life, and for their own suffering and death.

In turn, explicit death-shaming has sedimented down into a broader sense of inevitability around deaths that might otherwise be shocking or difficult to ignore. In his work on race, class and slow death in COVID-19, Tony Sandset uses Achille Mbembe's concept of necropolitics to question 'under what conditions do we accept that some lives will end and others will be saved under a pandemic? What kind of power structures allow certain lives to be conceptualized as acceptable deaths?' (Mbembe, 2019; Sandset, 2021: 1415). The machinery of shame, we argue, has been a vital component of necropolitics in the modern world; COVID-19 provides a case study in how shamed behaviour is used to legitimise (and desensitise publics to) specific instances of death, shifting responsibility from the political to the personal. For Sandset, necropolitics dictates who gets to live and die, but also who gets to be grieved; whose deaths are met with outrage and whose are met with acceptance (Sandset, 2021: 1415–1416). Throughout the coronavirus pandemic, people who are ageing, disabled, chronically ill or belong to ethnic minorities have been frequently figured as expendable (Sparke and Williams, 2022). Through the shame attached to vaccine hesitancy and refusal, unvaccinated people have been similarly constructed as a shamed and expendable group, governing how and whether their deaths are publicly grieved, ridiculed or forgotten, and enabling political decisions (such as the complete de-escalation of protective measures) which expose them to harm. A return to 'business as usual' – with relatively high mortality rates continuing – has rested in part on a high proportion of deaths being thought to occur among people who have 'failed to comply' with vaccination. These are shamed deaths, and so are politically and publicly bearable.

In this chapter, we examine recent discourses on vaccine hesitancy, death and dying through a 'shame lens' (Dolezal and Gibson, 2022). Our 2023 book, *COVID-19 and Shame: Political Emotions and Public Health in the UK*, considers the workings of shame in a series of contexts, narratives and experiences, primarily confined to 2020, the first year of the COVID-19 pandemic (Cooper et al., 2023). The present chapter builds on this work by turning its shame lens on a different but related phenomenon that gathered momentum in 2021 with the advent of mass vaccination programmes in some countries. To begin with, we situate our argument within longer histories of shame, public health and vaccination. This context depended upon an as-yet-unresolved tension between shame as a public health problem and its use as a public health tool, which raises important questions over communication and emotional leverage. Public health narratives which set out to shame vaccine-hesitant populations play a decisive role in framing and justifying instances of shaming in other contexts and situations.

We then explore the impact of online eruptions of shame around vaccine refusal and 'hesitancy'. We argue that shaming over vaccination status has harmed both its recipients and their likelihood of vaccine uptake, and represents an unnecessary barrier to healthy choices where many such barriers exist already. Lower vaccination rates are correlated to people with long experiences of structural abandonment and shaming, and often a justified mistrust of political and medical systems. Vaccine shame has to be understood as a problem of health inequalities more broadly, with considerable potential to heighten and exacerbate entrenched processes of disparity and discrimination (Scambler, 2020). Conscious decisions over where, how and what to communicate have been key to these processes, with the myth of 'hard to reach' populations deflecting shame from institutions with a responsibility to communicate effectively.

Finally, we focus on the specific confluence of vaccine hesitancy, 'vaxenfreude', the spectacle of taking joy in the illness or loss of vaccine- or COVID-deniers, and shameful death. Future crises, we suggest, will introduce novel (if historically framed and inflected) relationships between shame and death, just like this one. Critical reflection on the COVID-19 pandemic allows us to anticipate some of the contexts and processes which are likely to condition how and where they land, offering a conceptual framework which can be adapted to emergencies which are (at least partially) unforeseeable at the time of writing.

Shame and COVID-19

Shame is a negative self-conscious emotion that results from apprehensions of having been deemed to have transgressed or broken a social rule or norm, or from being judged to be otherwise flawed or compromised. Shame is always historically embedded and politically inflected, with what is considered 'shameful' deeply contingent on socio-cultural and political norms. The emotion is profoundly significant for understanding subjectivity, identity and social relations, and is inextricably tangled with structures, values and ideologies (Dolezal, 2015; Lewis, 1992; Lynd, 1958; Zahavi, 2014). For Erving Goffman, shame is a ubiquitous experience, and an ever-present possibility in almost all human interactions. While relatively few lives are shaped in their entirety by the active experience of shame, almost all are shaped by shame avoidance, insofar as the possibility for shame is an unspoken boundary that delimits what is 'appropriate', 'acceptable', 'proper' or 'normal'. Shame therefore plays a central role in the maintenance, and sometimes policing, of social norms (Goffman, 1959). It is an inevitable part of human experience and social relations. However, too much shame can be unhealthy, oppressive and potentially toxic (Bradshaw, 2005; Sanderson, 2015). Instead of facilitating personal, moral and social growth, excessive shame can be destructive, leading to a diminished personal and relational existence (DeYoung, 2015; Harris-Perry, 2011; Nathanson, 1992; Pattison, 2000). Importantly, shame does not have to be consciously or explicitly accepted by the subject – in the sense of agreement that an action, belief or identity is shame-worthy – to cause considerable harm.

With the potential to become a deeply negative phenomenon, shame can be a powerful political emotion, mobilised to manipulate, coerce and motivate others. Often, those with high levels of social power attempt to incite shame, through deliberate acts of *shaming*, for purposes of control, conformity, punishment or exclusion (Fischer, 2018). Shaming, as Martha Nussbaum notes, is a stigmatising judgement, where an individual or a group judges and condemns another for transgressing or failing to live up to an ideal or norm that is shared by a community, by society or by a cultural or political grouping (Nussbaum, 2004: 184–186). As shame carries with it the threat of losing social bonds and feeling rejected or ostracised from one's social group, shaming is a powerful means to motivate conformity to particular norms, rules, expectations or standards. In addition, shaming is also a means to publicly perform one's values and standards, or those of one's social grouping (Creed et al., 2014: 280). In judicial and formal punitive contexts (such as legal judgements and law enforcement), shaming is suggested to serve a pro-social function; it is often assumed that shaming will lead to recognition that one has fallen short of the standards of one's community and then subsequently motivate individuals to make positive changes to bring themselves back in line with the community's values, norms and mores.

Keying into cultural, relational and social concerns regarding belonging, embodied connection, reputation and status, intentional uses of shaming can punish, isolate, oppress, disadvantage or marginalise individuals, groups or populations. Over the last 50 years, the individualising logics of neoliberalism have shifted and intensified what we might call systemic shame, or shame which moves beyond the peculiarities of interpersonal situations and relationships. The convergence between public health imperatives and what Stuart Hall and Alan O'Shea term the 'structural consequences' of neoliberalism, 'the individualisation of everyone, the privatisation of public troubles and the requirement to make competitive choices at every turn', heightens the burden of shame on those unable to fit the ideal of the healthy, self-actualising neoliberal subject (Hall and O'Shea, 2013: 12). The (altered) rubrics of public health work continue to demand attention to determinants of health and illness, at the same time as neoliberal logic situates such determinants with individual decisions rather than structural contexts and processes (Spratt, 2021: 2). For Graham Scambler, the 'weaponisation' of stigma under financial capitalism has 'led to a political "skewing" of social norms of shame and blame', holding people with disabilities and chronic ill-health 'progressively more "personally responsible" for their impairments, shifting [them] in the process from "rejects" to "abjects"' (Scambler, 2018: 777, 780). Imogen Tyler explains how stigma is 'purposefully crafted as a strategy of government, in ways that often deliberately seek to foment and accentuate inequalities and injustices'. 'Ordinary' people, including those from shamed groups, are conscripted into this machinery, helping to spread or perpetuate shame and acting against their own interests in the process (Tyler, 2020: 18).

The coronavirus pandemic created new contexts for shame and shaming, but these largely followed well-travelled – if not wholly predictable – routes, frequently accruing around groups with longer histories of being subject to shame, fear and suspicion, often (but not always) in respect to the spread of disease. At times encouraged by high-profile politicians, people cast shame at members of groups perceived to be particularly infectious – such as medical professionals and people of Asian backgrounds – and policed the behaviour, actions and intentions of others through public censure and opprobrium, often on social media (Dolezal et al., 2021; Fang and Liu, 2021; Marcus, 2020; Tait, 2020). Frequently, experiences of shaming have been cumulative and intersectional, cutting deepest where people and groups with long experiences of being publicly shamed become tangled in newer dynamics of viral shaming (Mayer and Vanderheiden, 2021: 8). The core component of neoliberal shaming, the sleight of hand by which systemic problems are pinned on individual actors, has been extended and heightened over the course of the pandemic.

In the UK, the government repeatedly set out to deflect shame from both their own poor handling of the immediate crisis, and their long complicity in the raft of endemic problems which COVID-19 brought into sharper focus; including the 'slow death' of stark health inequalities among racialised communities (Sandset, 2021: 1412; see also Berlant, 2007). Unsatisfactory rates of infection and death were blamed on individuals ignoring advice, breaking rules, burdening the UK's National Health Service (NHS) with complications, or not using their 'common sense', frequently demonising groups who were already socially disadvantaged (Cooper, 2021; Dolezal and Spratt, 2023). Public health policy and messaging actively directed shame towards the populations it targeted, drawing on some of the most harmful traditions in its history (Cooper et al., 2023).

Public health and vaccine hesitancy

Public health interventions and communications have significant narrative power, telling stories about causation which can puncture or inflame political and public atmospheres around shaming. Where public health work takes explicit steps to destigmatise health challenges or mitigate against the ill-effects of shame, this can be decisive in reducing shame on a broad cultural level. Conversely, where shame is deliberately or unwittingly produced in pursuit of public health objectives, this helps to legitimise other – and perhaps more extreme – iterations of shame and shaming. One particularly visible example of the effects of public health messaging in producing shame can be seen in the UK Government's 2020 'better health' campaign, which explicitly positioned people with excess weight as making poor lifestyle choices and burdening the NHS (Dolezal and Spratt, 2023). In this instance, well-worn patterns of body shaming in public health were adapted to the COVID-19 context, even as the pandemic placed heightened constraints on the pursuit and maintenance of a 'healthy' weight.

Shame and shaming have inflected much of the public discourse around vaccine hesitancy. A high-profile Twitter debate between Brené Brown and Naomi Klein in May 2021 on the efficacy of shaming in relation to COVID-19 vaccines highlighted some of the core concerns regarding the use of shaming to motivate individuals to take up vaccines, as opposed to the use of shaming to motivate governments to make vaccines more widely available. Shaming, Brené Brown argues, 'is a tool of oppression – it will never be a tool for social justice (or public health)' (quoted in Golafshani, 2022: n.p.). Indeed, the relationship between vaccine hesitancy and shame must be understood in light of the long history, and ongoing ambivalence, regarding the use of shame and shaming within public health. Public health initiatives often use implicit, and sometimes even explicit, shaming as a means to motivate individual or social change in the service of public health. However, the use of shaming is also a highly contested and much criticised practice. Those who defend the use of shame as a tool for positive change point to the fact that it sometimes works; by appealing to an audience's sense of shame around particular behaviours or practices, it has been possible to effect a shift in habits among some of those targeted (Duong, 2021).

However, there is strong evidence in the global public health literature that campaigns using shame, blame or stigma to motivate individuals are often counter-productive. These shame campaigns can easily compound or exacerbate negative health outcomes and ill health, especially for members of groups that are already vulnerable, marginalised or living with health inequalities. As Robert Walker argues, 'explicit shame is best avoided as its effects are unpredictable' (Walker, 2014: 52). Reliably predicting how shaming will affect an individual or group is difficult. It seems clear, however, that shaming is more likely to harm communities and individuals that already have long experiences of public and structural shame; for instance, those who live in poverty, live with chronic illness, obesity or mental ill health, or who are minoritised or marginalised in other ways. Shaming also runs the risk of eliciting defensive responses and decreasing receptivity to public health advice, as recipients reject shame and lose trust in institutions and experts (Brewis and Wutich, 2019a). Reviewing evidence from global public health campaigns on hygiene, obesity and mental illness, the medical anthropologists Alexandra Brewis and Amber Wutich concluded that 'shame in all its forms needs to be removed from the public health tool kit, because it too easily misfires' (Brewis and Wutich, 2019b: 188).

This fundamental tension in how public health systems approach shame has been reflected in research on vaccination status. A 2017 article in the *Journal of Law, Medicine & Ethics*, 'Shaming vaccine refusal', set out to 'weigh the potential harms' of 'shaming (also known as denormalizing) vaccine refusal, creating or reinforcing social norms against vaccine refusal by characterizing it as a selfish act based on fears unsupported by facts' (Silverman and Wiley, 2017: 570). Although the authors, Ross Silverman and Lindsay Wiley, acknowledged that shame was a difficult and potentially counter-productive emotion with serious consequences, they concluded that 'refusal of vaccines is not so all-encompassing [as, for example, severe mental illness] and shaming vaccine refusal is not so identity spoiling as to be inescapable'; it offered a form of temporary stigmatisation that could be left behind by those marked out. Indeed, such a transformation – from fleeting shame to social reintegration – was the crux of the mechanism by which a modest application of shame effected behavioural change (Silverman and Wiley, 2017: 577). Shaming public health strategies, Silverman and Wiley noted, 'do not yet cross the line into the harsh social shaming that some private commentators have adopted' (Silverman and Wiley, 2017: 578).

Setting aside the point that shaming public health messages create fertile conditions for more overtly unpalatable scenes of shame, Silverman and Wiley's characterisation of vaccine shame as a shallow or fleeting phenomenon has not been borne out by subsequent events. As a pandemic with vast political, social and cultural repercussions, COVID-19 allowed for the mobilisation of discourses on national duty which, while not new, have saturated everyday life to an arguably distinctive extent (Kohlt, 2020). In this atmosphere of hyper-visibility, judgement and surveillance over vaccine decisions, hesitancy has been weighted in ways that have the potential for long-lasting changes to identity, feelings of shame and loss of trust in medical and political systems.

The 'line' that Silverman and Wiley drew between public health rhetoric and the shaming methods deployed by private actors has also at times been a confection. In a 2021 article published in *Vaccine*, the journal of the Japanese Society for Vaccinology, an interdisciplinary team of Yale academics explored the effects of what they termed 'persuasive messaging to increase COVID-19 vaccine uptake intentions' (James et al., 2021). Testing a series of narratives on vaccination and vaccine refusal for their efficacy in convincing participants to accept the vaccine, they argued that 'effective public health messages would also increase people's willingness to encourage those close to them to vaccinate and to hold negative judgments of those who do not vaccinate' (James et al., 2021: 7159). Two of the three most effective narratives trialled, or what the authors described as 'the most promising messages', were 'Not Bravery' and 'Community Interest + Embarrassment'. These titles become clearer when their corresponding messages are reproduced:

> Community Interest + Embarrassment: Imagine how embarrassed and ashamed you will be if you choose not to get vaccinated and spread COVID-19 to someone you care about.
>
> Not Bravery: People who refuse to get vaccinated against COVID-19 when there is a vaccine available because they don't think they will get sick or aren't worried about it aren't brave, they are reckless. By not getting vaccinated, you risk the health of your family, friends, and community. There is nothing attractive and independent-minded about ignoring public health guidance to get the COVID-19 vaccine. (James et al., 2021: 7160)

This deployment of shaming to reduce vaccine hesitancy clearly went beyond chasing the transitory shame attached to a perceived bad judgement call. This kind of shame –directed explicitly towards the person behind the behaviour – is sticky and difficult, belittling and damaging. While the logic behind this messaging is that saturating the recipient in shame will cause their decision to not be vaccinated to become socially untenable, theorisations of both shame and vaccine refusal suggest the opposite is just as (if not more) likely. Shame can cause the shamed party to reject the basis (ideas, evidence, authority, ideology) on which they were shamed, hardening what might have otherwise been a passing opinion or habit. Uses of shame to create behavioural change can never fully anticipate what form shame avoidance might take; permanently losing trust in the source of the message, for example, or closer personal identification with the object of shaming (Golafshani, 2022). Shame is an identity-forming emotion, not a quick behavioural fix. Likewise, Elisa Sobo encourages us to comprehend vaccine refusal as an act of becoming. Although it 'generally entails various important critiques (of the political economy, biomedicine, etc.)', she argues, it is also 'a highly social act—an act that, each time it is undertaken, reinforces social belonging by vitalizing community ties' (Sobo, 2016: 345). In her work on the parents of autistic children, Chloe Silverman has also demonstrated how anti-vaccination sentiment can be crucial to self-perceptions of 'good parenting', with scepticism over scientific evidence viewed as a kind of 'moral imperative' (Silverman, 2012: 225). These kinds of complex emotional and relational stakes in vaccine refusal are not fertile ground for communications which pivot on shame. If public health messages on COVID-19 vaccination seek to create a brief and clarifying experience of shame, then this is unlikely to land in the expected way. Instead, they risk harms of a longer duration, with complex repercussions for health; or, in the worst case, a shamed death. In a context where vaccine hesitancy is widely shamed, dying with COVID-19 fixes shame securely in time, obviating the possibility of recantation or return.

'Vaxenfreude' and the shameful death

In the public health messages discussed above, the 'vaccine hesitant', here a homogeneous and undifferentiated mass defined only by hesitation or refusal, were not just recipients of communications which set out to shame them into behavioural change. In the assertion that 'effective public health messages would also increase people's willingness to … hold negative judgments of those who do not vaccinate', unvaccinated people became the intentional victims of a broader project of affective engineering (James et al., 2021: 7159). Encouragements to vaccinate, in this sense, pivoted explicitly on the creation of a shamed out-group, going hand-in-hand with encouragements to negatively value those who declined or demurred. The use of shame as a tool of persuasion carries the seeds of a deeper erosion of sympathy, shading into ridicule and scorn; when shaming tactics fail to result in the desired-for change, the shame that they deploy does not simply dissipate easily or without harm. In the case of vaccine shaming, it resulted in a phenomenon which has been usefully termed 'vaxenfreude', in which any claim to a generative use of shame was largely abandoned.

A contraction of 'vaccine' or 'vaccination' and the widely-known German word 'schadenfreude', the feeling of taking joy in the pain or difficulty of another, vaxenfreude joined a growing list of what Amanda Roig-Marín describes as 'coroneologisms', new and resonant words thrown up by experiences of the coronavirus pandemic (Roig-Marín, 2021). In other work, we have discussed the origins, use and consequences of the term 'covidiot' as a means of casting shame (Cooper et al., 2023). Brought to prominence in September 2021 by Tyler Weyant, an editor at the US politics website POLITICO, 'vaxenfreude' denoted 'the joy the vaccinated feel when the unvaccinated get COVID-19'. Weyant named vaxenfreude to write against it; he described it as a 'dark spirit', rooted in smugness and judgementalism, a problem which underlined the disintegration of collective empathy and community spirit supposedly present at the beginning of the pandemic (Weyant, 2021: n.p.). Indeed, the social psychologist Colin Leach has argued that gloating and schadenfreude are exacerbated as a result of political polarisation: 'When it's a serious rivalry, which is what politics is these days, it's not just taking a little pleasure in somebody's misfortune … it's seeing your enemies suffer because of what they believe. This is the sweetest justice, and that's partly why it's so satisfying to the other side' (quoted by Levin, 2021: n.p.).

The day after Weyant coined 'vaxenfreude', an article in *The Week* connected it specifically with shame and death, reproducing the testimony of a funeral director in Pennsylvania who reported that families were requesting that COVID-19 be left off death notices (Weber, 2021). Drawing heavily on Weyant's piece and an episode of the National Public Radio (NPR) podcast *All Things Considered*, the article cited research on grief undertaken by Ken Doka, Senior Vice President of the Hospice Foundation of America. For Doka, specific kinds of death, and their subsequent mourning by relatives and friends – are 'disenfranchised', a process through which death is 'tinged with a supposed moral failure and mourners fear judgment from others' (Sholtis, 2021: n.p.). Where mass vaccination gathered momentum, dying with COVID-19 came to be qualified by vaccine status, inflecting political and cultural stories around death – as well as instances of actual death – with varying degrees of grievability.

A measure of this grievability can be taken in the emergence of social media forums that aimed to shame people across the scepticism spectrum. The r/HermanCainAward subreddit (dedicated section of the user-driven website Reddit), named after a Republican politician who died of COVID-19 after opposing masking mandates), the *Sorry*AntiVaxxer.com website and the @CovidiotDeaths Twitter handle documented cases of people 'who made public declaration of their anti-mask, anti-vax, or Covid-hoax views, followed by admission to hospital for Covid'.[1] Using a combination of posts and memes posted to social media, contributors would reconstruct the decisions of their targets into narratives, complete with a developed dramatic irony that found an eager and vindictive readership. The sites were premised on the idea that these hospitalisations or deaths were deserved, and the people they involved were stupid. In this sense, they contributed to a growing sense that to die of COVID when unvaccinated was to die a shameful death. According to Allan Kellehear, such a death involves '[d]ying too soon and from a stigmatising disease, or taking so long to die when you are old so that you become confused, unmanageable and unrecognisable to friends or other professionals ... styles of dying that are both uncertain, ambiguous and a spoiled activity for all participants involved'. Parallels can be seen in the shame attached by homophobic political and medical responses to dying with acquired immunodeficiency virus (AIDS), or the 'sympathy difference' in dying with cancers widely understood to be products of lifestyle choices (Kellehear, 2007: 214). At face value, the shaming perpetrated in forums like r/HermanCainAward adds a conditional to the general stigma associated with catching COVID-19. If someone has chosen not to get vaccinated, then this choice spoils their 'style of dying' and they deserve the opprobrium of others.

Under this new rubric, those who had died having refused the vaccine were deemed less grievable than those who died despite receiving it or before it was offered. The vaccinated/not-yet-vaccinated death fulfilled a narrative arc in which the dead person could usually be straightforwardly construed as the victim (of course, this is complicated somewhat by other iterations of culpability and shaming over pandemic behaviour or pre-existing health). Conversely, the vaccine refuser is the knowing architect of their own misfortune, responsible for their own fate and tarnished further by the act of having exposed others to either direct viral harm or the myriad challenges of an ongoing pandemic. Narratives that seek to shame the unvaccinated, however, seldom bother to complicate matters by considering the conditions under which 'personal choice' is exercised, or by distinguishing between homogenising characterisations of the 'anti-vaxxer'. Individual choice is imagined to be paramount. And yet, as other scenes of the pandemic demonstrated, individual choice is always constrained by circumstance; the rationale of the person concerned with side effects is conflated with that of someone who denies the severity of the disease, or the vocal denier is conflated with the quiet abstainer. More than simply 'dying too soon and from a stigmatising disease', dying while unvaccinated was a shameful death because the dead person had chosen this for themselves, and this choice had consequences for other people.

Studies that explicitly set out to understand vaccine hesitancy, however, emphasise the complexity of factors and contexts which frame and govern 'individual' decisions to accept vaccines. 2021 research into hesitancy over childhood vaccines in the Philippines (with COVID-19 as the backdrop but not the focus) used spoken testimonies from parents to demonstrate a raft of interconnected barriers to vaccination. The team divided these into 'individual barriers', including 'perceived lack of information', conflicting religious or cultural beliefs, 'competing time demands' and the traumatic fallout from a historic dengue fever vaccine controversy; 'interpersonal and community barriers', which factored in opposition to vaccines from household heads, community leaders and neighbours; 'health system barriers', including lack of trust and logistical problems (such as waiting times and appointment scheduling); and 'superstructural barriers', including poor or non-existent access to transport, bad weather and COVID-19 (Landicho-Guevarra et al., 2021: 6). Carlos Amato's cartoon did at least represent multiple reasons for refusal, but they were all relegated to the realm of decontextualised choice; contrary and opinionated people who thought they knew better, but were wrong. This is hardly what emerges here, or in any detailed and thoughtful work on refusal and hesitancy.

In addition, COVID-19 vaccination has not been a demographically consistent phenomenon. Already giving the lie to easy attributions of blame and shame, a complex nexus of barriers and demotivating factors has been complicated further by clear disparities in vaccine uptake along pre-existing lines of marginalisation and exclusion, particularly (but not exclusively) in terms of experiences of structural racism. Multiple studies in the UK have established that members of racialised groups have been more likely to be vaccine hesitant than those who identify as white British, often by a considerable margin. This point is well documented, as are the factors which are used to explain it: heightened barriers to access; higher perceptions of risk; decreased levels of confidence and trust in medical systems, politicians and the vaccines themselves; and culturally specific factors such as travel restrictions or concern over specific ingredients (Chaudhuri et al., 2022; Gong, 2022; Kasstan, 2021; Scientific Advisory Group on Emergencies, 2020; Woolf et al., 2021). These factors, the studies note, are also significant in understanding the greater hesitancy of groups whose members are otherwise structurally disadvantaged.

Behind this sanitising language, however, is a series of deeper historical challenges. The problem of 'access' misconstrues a generalised system of racist discrimination; the problem of 'trust' elides long histories of harm and neglect in medical research and practice (Phiri et al., 2021: 2–3; see also Limb, 2021). Vaccine hesitancy among members of racialised minorities can be understood as yet another product of structural racism, joining the 'slow death' of pre-existing health inequalities and the necropolitics of sanctioned exposure to COVID-19, in dictating who gets to live or die, and which deaths are grieved or accepted (Ford, 2020; ONS, 2022; Qureshi et al., 2022; Sparke and Williams, 2022). Indeed, they are all parts of the same equation. In a pandemic where ethnic minorities have been repeatedly shamed both for supposedly spreading the virus and for dying from it in greater numbers, the undifferentiated shaming of the vaccine hesitant has the effect of 'heaping blame on shame' (Scambler, 2020: 79).

Writing on the 'acceptability' of specific kinds of pandemic death, Sandset cites a short passage taken from Judith Butler's 2006 work, *Precarious Life: The Powers of Mourning and Violence*. In it, Butler suggests that the 'differential allocation of grievability ... operates to produce and maintain certain exclusionary concepts of who is normatively human'. Sandset develops this point into an argument over what he terms the 'state of acceptance', or 'how we have come to accept that certain lives will be more vulnerable' (Butler, 2006: x; Sandset, 2021: 1415). Rather than the 'exceptional state[s] of emergency' explored by Mbembe in his original formulation of necropolitics, Sandset theorises acceptance as the legitimising affect of necropower (Sandset, 2021: 1415). Vaccine shaming, we argue, has been a crucial component of political and public acceptance over continued deaths from COVID-19 – for example, in the emergence of terms such as 'pandemic of the unvaccinated' (Zamir and Gillis, 2023) – allowing government actions to expose both vaccinated and unvaccinated people to ongoing harms. This represented a crucial development of the shaming narratives which emerged in the early stages of the pandemic, in which shame over high rates of infection and death were deflected away from the state and towards the contravention of public health guidance, a lack of common sense, and pre-existing conditions and habits (such as poor diet and insufficient exercise) which made serious or fatal illness more likely. These had always been attempts at saving face, mobilised to draw the focus away from acute and chronic political and ethical failures (Cooper et al., 2023).

The wide celebration of the vaccine as a magic bullet, eclipsing complementary measures organised around behaviour, access to spaces or hygiene, greatly raised the (already considerable) stakes on individual dissent (Farrar, 2020). In framing vaccination programmes as a 'race against the virus', public health rhetoric posed even temporary hesitation as a loaded and potentially shameful act (Channel 4, 2020; Durbin, 2021). A small series of acts of refusal, deferment or omission became life- and death-defining, as in the reproduction of anti-vaccine or vaccine-sceptical social media posts as a kind of extended suicide note (Bruenig, 2021). Even in far less overtly shaming discourses, unvaccinated deaths have been systematically unmoored from their deeper contexts. With confusion persisting over mortality rates by vaccine status, and early disparities increasingly more difficult to separate cleanly, the existence of a significant number of deaths which are plausibly (within individualising logics of blame and shame) the fault of the deceased has the effect of contributing to a state of acceptance over all continuing COVID-19 deaths. The closest parallel this phenomenon has is the fallacy that COVID-19 'only' has serious effects on the old, disabled or chronically ill. Although it is clear that this notion of expendability enclosed significant components of shame, the problem of direct blame was mostly absent from the equation, even as specific lives were explicitly discarded and devalued (Aronson, 2020; Pring, 2021). In the case of the unvaccinated, the machinery of shame around vaccine hesitancy and refusal shifted them into the necropolitical zone of acceptable death. This process had consequences for the vaccinated as well as the unvaccinated dead, skewing perceptions of grievability even around those who, by the pro-vaccination standards of public health, had done everything right.

How did shaming discourses around vaccine hesitancy inflect experiences of dying? As Doka's notion of disenfranchised death (cited in Sholtis, 2021: n.p.) suggests, the cultural and political framing of specific experiences of dying and grief has significant repercussions for how these processes are lived. Kellehear notes how shame is internalised by sufferers in the (often long and drawn-out) process of dying, making the experience 'painfully worse than the physical and medical settings ruthlessly dictate'; cathartic experiences of grief, both individually and collectively, are further conditioned by the shame dynamics which surround the cause and manner of death (Kellehear, 2007: 218). A recent Lancet Commission report has explored and (re)asserted the need to properly value death and dying; the extreme circumstances of the pandemic have taken us even further away from anything vaguely recognisable as a 'good death' (Sallnow et al., 2022). People have died in jarring and abject ways: before they grew old, on ventilators, and on video calls with relatives (Weir, 2020). The shame that accrued around dying from COVID-19 – let alone dying unvaccinated from COVID-19 – worked to further exclude those left behind from a relational experience of mourning, isolating them further in their grief.

The concept of shameful death, here, can only take us so far. While the dying might experience shame related to their decisions, once they are dead it can only be those who live on who can experience shame *on their behalf*. Far from being a metaphysical thought-experiment, there were numerous cases of people being overwhelmed with difficult emotions when they found relatives listed as r/HermanCain awardees or *Sorry*AntiVaxxer.com targets (Judkis, 2021). They also produced empathy with the shamed party. In a *Slate* article in September 2021, Lili Loofbourow explored the 'unbelievable grimness' of the r/HermanCainAward subreddit. Moving beyond the superficial critique of 'death-shaming' present in similar commentary, Loofbourow noted that it made room for something largely absent elsewhere, in the form of a detailed and extensive record of what it's like to die with COVID-19: 'what hundreds of stories about deaths told through mean-spirited screenshots reveal is that the disease—when it gets bad—is worse than even the most pro-vax person really understood'. Loofbourow conceptualised the r/HermanCainAward as an 'anti-persuasive' space, a characteristic which – paradoxically – underpinned the only power it had to persuade (Loofbourow, 2021: n.p.).

This returns us to one of the central arguments behind our rejection of shame as a public health tool, and criticism of discourses which encourage it in wider public behaviour; it is impossible to determine exactly how and where it will land, and precisely what effects it will have. While the act of shaming can be read as an attempt to assert control, it is also an act of unintentional relinquishing, of releasing dangerous emotions into the wild. Although our discussion of shame and death has been largely confined to the problem of vaccine hesitancy in the COVID-19 pandemic, the lessons we draw – about how shame in public health can help to frame harmful eruptions of public shaming, and how these can enter into feedback loops with the politics of dying and grief – will continue to resonate in future crises, whether economic, political, military, viral or environmental. While neoliberal logics frame discourses on (and experiences of) choice, safety, health and illness, some deaths will be freighted with shame, devalued and subject to political and cultural acceptance; regrettable but not grievable, at least not in the sense defined by Butler (2006). If crises can also be opportunities, critical reflection on the contexts and harms of shame during COVID-19 can better equip us to understand how they might play out next.

Note

1 u/HubrisAndScandals, 'r/HermanCainAward', Reddit. Available at: www.reddit.com/r/HermanCainAward/ (accessed 4 July 2022).

References

Amato, Carlos (2021), Grave mistakes, New Frame, 24 August. Available at: www.newframe.com/cartoon-grave-mistakes/

Aronson, Louise (2020), 'COVID-19 kills only old people'. Only?, New York Times, 22 March. Available at: www.nytimes.com/2020/03/22/opinion/coronavirus-elderly.html

Berlant, Lauren (2007), Slow death (sovereignty, obesity, lateral agency). Critical Inquiry, 33(4), 754–780. https://doi.org/10.1086/521568

Bradshaw, John (2005), Healing the Shame That Binds You. Deerfield Beach, FL: Health Communications, Inc.

Brewis, Alexandra and Wutich, Amber (2019a), Why we should never do it: Stigma as a behaviour change tool in global health. BMJ Global Health, 4, e001911. https://doi.org/10.1136/bmjgh-2019-001911

Brewis, Alexandra and Wutich, Amber (2019b), Lazy, Crazy and Disgusting: Stigma and the Undoing of Global Health. Baltimore, MD: Johns Hopkins University Press.

Bruenig, Elizabeth (2021), Stop death shaming: Mocking the unvaccinated dead does not save lives, The Atlantic, 2 September. Available at: www.theatlantic.com/ideas/archive/2021/09/stop-death-shaming/619939/

Butler, Judith (2006), Precarious Life: The Powers of Mourning and Violence. London: Verso Books.

Channel 4. (2020), Race against the virus: Hunt for a vaccine', 3 August.

Chaudhuri, K., Chakrabarti, A., Chandan, J. S., et al. (2022), COVID-19 vaccine hesitancy in the UK: A longitudinal household cross-sectional study. BMC Public Health, 22, Article no. 104. Available at: https://doi.org/10.1186/s12889-021-12472-3

Cooper, Fred (2021), Shame, common sense and COVID-19: Notes from mass observation, blog post, Shame and Medicine, 14 December. Available at: https://shameandmedicine.org/shame-common-sense-and-COVID-19-notes-from-mass-observation/

Cooper, Fred, Dolezal, Luna and Rose, Arthur (2023), *COVID-19 and Shame: Political Emotions and Public Health in the UK*. London: Bloomsbury.

Creed, W. E. Douglas, Hudson, B. A., Okhuysen, G. A., et al. (2014), Swimming in a sea of shame: Incorporating emotion into explanations of institutional reproduction and change. *Academy of Management Review*, 39(3), 275–301.

DeYoung, Patricia A. (2015), *Understanding and Treating Chronic Shame: A Relational/Neurobiological Approach*. London: Routledge.

Dolezal, Luna (2015), *The Body and Shame: Phenomenology, Feminism and the Socially Shaped Body*. Lanham, MD: Lexington Books.

Dolezal, Luna, Rose, Arthur and Cooper, Fred (2021), COVID-19, online shaming, and health-care professionals. *Lancet*, 398, 482–483.

Dolezal, Luna and Gibson, Matthew (2022), Beyond a trauma-informed approach and towards shame-sensitive practice. *Humanities and Social Sciences Communications*, 9(214), 1–10.

Dolezal, Luna and Spratt, Tanisha (2023), Fat shaming under neoliberalism and COVID-19: Examining the UK's 'Tackling Obesity' campaign. *Sociology of Health and Illness*, 45(1), 3–18.

Duong, Diana (2021), Does shaming have a place in public health? *CMAJ: Canadian Medical Association Journal (Journal de l'Association medicale canadienne)*, 193(2), E59–E60. Available at: https://doi.org/10.1503/cmaj.1095910

Durbin, Adam (2021), Covid: UK in a 'race between virus and vaccine' over Omicron, says Sajid Javid, BBC News, 13 December. Available at: www.bbc.co.uk/news/uk-59634112

Fang, Nini and Liu, Shan-Jan Sarah (2021), Critical conversations: Being Yellow women in the time of COVID-19. *International Feminist Journal of Politics*, 23(2), 333–340.

Farrar, Jeremy (2020), Let's get real. No vaccine will work as if by magic, returning us to 'normal', *Guardian*, 6 September. Available at: www.theguardian.com/commentisfree/2020/sep/06/lets-get-real-no-vaccine-will-work-as-if-by-magic-returning-us-to-normal

Fischer, Clara (2018), Gender and the politics of shame: A twenty-first-century feminist shame theory. *Hypatia: A Journal of Feminist Philosophy*, 33(3), 372–383.

Ford, Megan (2020), Exclusive: BME nurses 'feel targeted' to work on COVID-19 wards, *Nursing Times*, 17 April. Available at: www.nursingtimes.net/news/coronavirus/exclusive-bme-nurses-feel-targeted-to-work-on-COVID-19-wards-17-04-2020/

Goffman, Erving (1959), *The Presentation of Self in Everyday Life*. Middlesex: Penguin Books.

Golafshani, Maryam (2022), Empathy and shame through critical phenomenology: The limits and possibilities of affective work in the case of COVID-19 vaccinations. *Journal of Evaluation in Clinical Practice*, 1–7. Published online ahead of print: https://doi.org/10.1111/jep.13761

Gong, Sarah (2022), Co-design and implement a COVID-19 vaccine uptake intervention within Chinese communities in England, Pandemic and Beyond Working Paper, 22 February. Available at: https://pandemicandbeyond.exeter.ac.uk/wp-content/uploads/2022/06/PB_Policy_Brief_Gong_Feb202232.pdf

Hall, Stuart and O'Shea, Alan (2013), Common-sense neoliberalism. *Soundings: A Journal of Politics and Culture*, 55, 8–24.

Harris-Perry, Melissa (2011), *Sister Citizen: Shame, Stereotypes and Black Women in America*. New Haven, CT and London: Yale University Press.

James, Erin K., Bokemper, S. E., Gerber, A. S., et al. (2021), Persuasive messaging to increase COVID-19 vaccine uptake intentions. *Vaccine*, 39, 7158–7165.

Judkis, Maura (2021), What do all these stories of vaccine denial deaths do to our sense of empathy?, *Washington Post*, 7 October. Available at: www.washingtonpost.com/lifestyle/style/anti-vaccine-deaths-no-sympathy/2021/10/06/779488e6-20ad-11ec-8200-5e3fd4c49f5e_story.html. Accessed 4 July 2022.

Kasstan, Ben (2021), Vaccines and vitriol: An anthropological commentary on vaccine hesitancy, decision-making and interventionism among religious minorities. *Anthropology & Medicine*, 28(4), 411–419. Available at: https://doi.org/10.1080/13648470.2020.1825618

Kellehear, Allan (2007), *A Social History of Dying*. Cambridge: Cambridge University Press.

Kohlt, Franziska (2020), 'Over by Christmas': The impact of war-metaphors and other science-religion narratives on science communication environments during the COVID-19 crisis, *SocArXiv Papers*, 10 November. Available at: https://doi.org/10.31235/osf.io/z5s6a

Kronbauer, Bob (2021), Opinion: 'I did my own research' skeleton wins Halloween, vancouverisawesome.com, 14 October. Available at: www.vancouverisawesome.com/opinion/i-did-my-own-research-meme-4513579

Landicho-Guevarra, Jhoys, Reñosa, Mark Donald C., Wachinger, Jonas, et al. (2021), Scared, powerless, insulted and embarrassed: Hesitancy towards vaccines among caregivers in Cavite Province, the Philippines. *BMJ Global Health*, 6, e006529. Available at: http://dx.doi.org/10.1136/bmjgh-2021-006529

Levin, Dan (2021), They died from COVID: Then the online attacks started, *New York Times*, 27 November. Available at: www.nytimes.com/2021/11/27/style/anti-vaccine-deaths-social-media.html

Lewis, Michael (1992), *Shame: The Exposed Self*. New York: The Free Press.

Limb, Matthew (2021), Disparity in maternal deaths because of ethnicity is 'unacceptable'. British Medical Journal, 372(152). Available at: https://doi.org/10.1136/bmj.n152

Loofbourow, Lili (2021), The unbelievable grimness of HermanCainAward, the subreddit that catalogs anti-vaxxer COVID deaths, Slate, 21 September. Available at: https://slate.com/technology/2021/09/hermancainaward-subreddit-antivaxxer-deaths-cataloged.html (accessed 4 July 2022).

Lynd, Helen (1958), *On Shame and the Search for Identity*. New York: Harcourt Brace.

Marcus, Julia (2020), Quarantine fatigue is real, *Atlantic*, 11 May. Available at: www.theatlantic.com/ideas/archive/2020/05/quarantine-fatigue-real-and-shaming-people-wont-help/611482/

Mayer, C. and Vanderheiden, E. (2021), Transforming shame in the pandemic: An international study. *Frontiers in Psychology*, 14(12), 641076. doi: 10.3389/fpsyg.2021.641076

Mbembe, Achille (2019), *Necropolitics*. Durham, NC: Duke University Press.

Nathanson, Donald (1992), *Shame and Pride: Affect, Sex and the Birth of the Self*. New York: W. W. Norton & Company.

Nussbaum, Martha (2004) *Hiding from Humanity: Disgust, Shame and the Law*. Princeton, NJ: Princeton University Press.

Office for National Statistics (ONS). (2022), Deaths involving COVID-19 by vaccination status, England: Deaths occurring between 1 January 2021 and 31 March 2022, 16 May. Available at: www.ons.gov.uk/peoplepopulationandcommunity/birthsdeathsandmarriages/deaths/bulletins/deathsinvolvingcovid19byvaccinationstatusengland/deathsoccurringbetween1january2021and31march2022

Pattison, Stephen (2000), *Shame: Theory, Therapy, Theology*. Cambridge: Cambridge University Press.

Phiri, Peter, et al. (2021), COVID-19 and Black, Asian, and Minority Ethnic communities: A complex relationship without just cause. *JMIR Public Health Surveillance*, 7(2). Available at: https://doi.org/10.2196/22581

Pring, John (2021), Pandemic 'has exposed the shadow of eugenics', TUC conference hears, Disability News Service, 11 March. Available at: www.disabilitynewsservice.com/pandemic-has-exposed-the-shadow-of-eugenics-tuc-conference-hears/

Qureshi, I., Gogoi, M., Wobi, F., et al. (2022), Healthcare workers from diverse ethnicities and their perceptions of risk and experiences of risk management during the COVID-19 pandemic: Qualitative insights from the United Kingdom-REACH Study. *Frontiers in Medicine*, 9(930904). doi: 10.3389/fmed.2022.930904

Roig-Marín, Amanda (2021), English-based Coroneologisms. *English Today*, 37(4), 193–195.

Sallnow, Libby, Smith, Richard, Ahmedzai, Sam H., et al. (2022), Report of the Lancet Commission on the Value of Death: Bringing death back into life. *Lancet*, 399(10327). Available at: https://doi.org/10.1016/S0140-6736(21)02314-X

Sanderson, Christine (2015), *Counselling Skills for Working with Shame*. London and Philadelphia: Jessica Kingsley Publishers.

Sandset, Tony (2021), The necropolitics of COVID-19: Race, class and slow death in an ongoing pandemic. *Global Public Health*, 16, 8–9.

Scambler, Graham (2018), Heaping blame on shame: 'Weaponising stigma' for neoliberal times. *The Sociological Review Monographs*, 66(4), 766–782.

Scambler, Graham (2020), *A Sociology of Shame and Blame: Insiders versus Outsiders*. Basingstoke: Palgrave Macmillan.

Scientific Advisory Group on Emergencies (UK). (2020). Factors influencing COVID-19 vaccine uptake among minority ethnic groups, 17 December. Available at: www.gov.uk/government/publications/factors-influencing-COVID-19-vaccine-uptake-among-minority-ethnic-groups-17-december-2020

Sholtis, Brett (2021), Attitudes around Covid can add even more pain and anger for those grieving loved ones, NPR, 7 September. Available at: www.npr.org/2021/09/07/1034926668/attitudes-around-covid-can-add-even-more-pain-and-anger-for-those-grieving-loved

Silverman, Chloe (2012), *Understanding Autism: Parents, Doctors, and the History of a Disorder*. Princeton, NJ: Princeton University Press.

Silverman, Ross D. and Wiley, Lindsay F. (2017), Shaming vaccine refusal. *The Journal of Law, Medicine & Ethics*, 45.

Sobo, Elisa J. (2016), Theorizing vaccine refusal: Through the looking glass. *Cultural Anthropology*, 31(3).

Sparke, Matthew and Williams, Owain David (2022), Neoliberal disease: COVID-19, co-pathogenesis and global health insecurities. *Environment and Planning A: Economy and Space*, 54(1), 15–32. doi: 10.1177/0308518X211048905

Spratt, Tanisha Jemma Rose (2021), Understanding 'fat shaming' in a neoliberal era: Performativity, healthism and the UK's 'obesity epidemic'. *Feminist Theory*, 24(1). Published online first: doi: 10.1177/14647001211048300

Tait, Amelia (2020), Pandemic shaming: Is it helping us to keep our distance?, *Guardian*, 4 April. Available at: www.theguardian.com/science/2020/apr/04/pandemic-shaming-is-it-helping-us-keep-our-distance

Tyler, Imogen (2020), *Stigma: The Machinery of Inequality*. London: Zed Books.

Walker, Robert (2014), *The Shame of Poverty*. Oxford: Oxford University Press.

Weber, Peter (2021), 'Vaxenfreude' and the shame around unvaccinated COVID-19 victims, The Week, 8 September. Available at: https://theweek.com/coronavirus/1004611/vaxenfreude-and-the-shame-around-unvaccinated-COVID-19-victims

Weir, Kirsten (2020), Grief and COVID-19: Saying goodbye in the age of physical distancing, American Psychological Association, 6 April. Available at: www.apa.org/topics/COVID-19/grief-distance

Weyant, Tyler (2021), The pandemic's new emotion: Vaxenfreude, POLITICO, 7 September. Available at: www.politico.com/newsletters/politico-nightly/2021/09/07/the-pandemics-new-emotion-vaxenfreude-494224

Woolf, Katherine, et al. (2021), Ethnic differences in SARS-CoV-2 vaccine hesitancy in United Kingdom healthcare workers: Results from the UK-REACH prospective nationwide cohort study. *Lancet Regional Health – Europe*, 9(100180).

Zahavi, Dan (2014), *Self and Other: Exploring Subjectivity, Empathy and Shame*. Oxford: Oxford University Press.

Zamir, E. and Gillis, P. (2023), The pandemic of the unvaccinated: A Covid-19 ethical dilemma. *Heart Lung*, 57, 292–294. Available at: www.ncbi.nlm.nih.gov/pmc/articles/PMC9420715/

Index

accessibility 22, 30, 32
affect 17–18, 25, 34
Age UK 137, 145–50
airborne transmission 21, 23, 25, 31
allocentric representation 46
Amato, Carlos 179
An Anti-Racist Health Service – A Manifesto for Change 167, 174
animation 24–5
   anthropomorphism 23, 29
   characters 22–4, 27, 29
   script writing 22, 24, 27, 30–3
autoethnography 141, 143–4

bacteria 16, 26
belonging 87, 100, 106
Black Lives Matter 172
Bristol Somali Youth Forum 19, 30
bus 16–35
   architecture 22–3, 28–30
   operators 20, 28
   users 20, 22, 26, 28, 33
Butler, Judith 193, 196

care 136, 140, 149, 151
career shock 115, 120–1
Caribbean African Health Network (CAHN) 161
chapter summaries 7–14
child to parent violence 149

cities
   connectedness and 87, 88, 89, 92, 93, 95, 101, 102, 103, 105, 106, 107
   disconnection in 87, 88, 9
   green-blue spaces in 100, 103, 107
   green spaces and 89, 95, 96, 107
   home-city geographies 87, 107
   local places 92, 108
   sociality and 94, 100, 101, 102, 105, 107
communication design 3
community 92, 93, 100, 103, 104, 105, 106, 107, 108
community engagement 114, 125
control 137–8, 145–8
   coercive 145–7
conviviality (urban) 88, 105
'coroneologisms' 189
crime data 139
Critical Race Theory 158–9

deafblindness 41–55
dis/ability 141
documentary of force 162–3
dwelling 87, 100, 105
dying 189–96
   as spoiled activity 190–1, 194–5

Index

egocentric representation 46
elder abuse 140
emotional labour 113, 124–6
emotions 114, 121, 124
    at/about museums 121, 124
    and work 125–7
epistemology 3–5
    see also knowledge
ethics 21, 28

face coverings 22, 31
film-making 25, 28, 33–4
    participatory 163–4
Floyd, George 172
furlough 117–18

gender-based violence 136–55
generation 137, 140, 148, 150
Gramsci, Antonio 163
grief 190
grievability 190–1, 196

haptic technology 46, 49
home 86–108
    see also 'stay home' directives
honour-based violence 149
humanities research 3–7
    methodologies 7, 14
    temporalities 6

immobilities 137, 142, 144, 147–8, 150
Independent SAGE 5
inequality 99, 104, 107
infection prevention 19, 21, 23–4, 27, 34–5
interdisciplinarity 33, 35
interspecies relatedness 16–17
Irish Linen Centre and Lisburn Museum 126

knowledge 18–19, 30, 32–3, 35
    see also epistemology

Latour, Bruno 2–3
lifecourse 140–1, 148
life writing 140–1
Liverpool 87, 90, 91, 93, 94, 97, 101, 103
lockdown 86, 88, 90, 91, 93, 94, 95, 102, 136–7, 144–5, 150
London 87, 90, 91, 93, 96, 103, 106
loneliness 93, 94, 95, 105

maps 90, 96, 97, 98
marginalisation 137
mass testing 1
Mbembe, Achille 180, 193
memory 124–5
microbial 16–35
    agency 16, 27
    aesthetics 18, 21, 23, 25–8
    communities 18, 23, 26–7, 29
    literacy 18, 25, 30, 34
    imaginary 20, 26, 34
        politics of 28–30
    relations 19, 23–4, 29
misogyny 136
more-than-human methods 17, 19, 22, 24, 27, 30, 33
mosques 103
multilingualism 28–9, 31, 34
museum 113–30
    activism 113
    closures 120–3
    collecting for 115, 126–7
    inequality 119–20
    local authority 122, 123, 128
    management 117
    purpose 115–16, 127
    relevance 114, 119, 121, 123, 128–9
    wellbeing 119–20, 122, 127
Museums Association 113–14, 118–19, 128
mutual aid 103, 104

National Health Service (NHS) 156–75, 184–5
National Lottery Heritage Fund 114

National Museums Northern Ireland 117, 122, 127
necropolitics 180, 192–4
neighbourhood/neighbourliness 86–108
neoliberalism 183–4
Northern Ireland Museums Council 114
Northern Ireland War Memorial 119, 123
Nursing and Midwifery Council 168

obstinate memory 162, 166, 174
older women 136–55
organic intellectuals 172
organisational adaptability 127–8

parks 95, 96, 97, 102, 103, 105, 107
personal protective equipment (PPE) 160
power 106
precarity 114, 118
public health 184–6, 187
    messaging 17, 19, 20–1, 23, 25, 27, 29, 30, 32–5
    and vaccination 186

qualitative methods 142–4

racism 105, 106, 156–75
Reddit
    r/HermanCainAward 195
religious faith 103, 104, 108
resilience 121–2

Scientific Advisory Group for Emergencies (SAGE) 5
shame 179–96
    and COVID-19 183–4
    theory 181–3
social distancing 42–3, 45
'stay home' directives 86, 87, 88, 90, 94, 106

'stay home' stories 87, 90, 107
stigma 20, 23, 183
storytelling 29–30, 34, 138, 141–3, 150

tests/testing 60–82
    community 61, 81
    design 60–82
    diagnostic 60–1, 63, 65–6, 77–8, 80–2
    diagrams 65, 68–70, 79
    home 61, 65, 81
        information 63, 65–6, 70–71, 82
        instructions 60–3, 65–6, 71–3, 77–82
        'quick guide' 73, 75–7
    lateral flow (LFT) 1–4, 9, 60–1, 66, 72–4, 78, 82
    point-of-use instruction toolkit 61, 66, 77–82
    rapid 60–1, 81
    usability 61–82
Third Cinema 158, 169
time/temporality 88
touch 41–55
    deprivation 42, 44–5
Tower Museum, Derry/Londonderry 114

United Kingdom (UK) government 1, 20, 25, 27, 30, 42, 54, 184
'better health' campaign 185

vaccine hesitancy 179–96
    complexity of 188, 191–2
    demographic disparities in 192–3
'vaxenfreude' 181, 188–9
visual mental imagery 44

walking 96, 97, 102
Workforce Race Equality Standard (WRES) 159

EU authorised representative for GPSR:
Easy Access System Europe, Mustamäe tee 50,
10621 Tallinn, Estonia
gpsr.requests@easproject.com